Preventive Medicine and Public Health

PreTest®
Self-Assessment
and Review

• NOTICE •

Medicine is an ever-changing science. As new research and clinical experience broaden our knowledge, changes in treatment and drug therapy are required. The editor and the publisher of this work have checked with sources believed to be reliable in their efforts to provide information that is complete and generally in accord with the standards accepted at the time of publication. However, in view of the possibility of human error or changes in medical sciences, neither the editor, nor the publisher, nor any other party who has been involved in the preparation or publication of this work warrants that the information contained herein is in every respect accurate or complete and they are not responsible for any errors or omissions or for the results obtained from use of such information. Readers are encouraged to confirm the information contained herein with other sources. For example and in particular, readers are advised to check the product information sheet included in the package of each drug they plan to administer to be certain that the information contained in this book is accurate and that changes have not been made in the recommended dose or in the contra-indications for administration. This recommendation is of particular importance in connection with new or infrequently used drugs.

Preventive Medicine and Public Health

PreTest® Self-Assessment and Review

Seventh Edition

Edited by

F. Douglas Scutchfield, M.D.
Professor and Director
Graduate School of Public Health
San Diego State University
San Diego, California

Contributions by

Jane F. Marystone, M.D.
Jacqueline H. Sedgewick, M.D.
Michael R. Snedecor, M.D., M.P.H.

Residents
University of California/San Diego State University
Preventive Medicine Residency
San Diego, California

McGraw-Hill, Inc.
Health Professions Division/PreTest® Series

New York   St. Louis   San Francisco   Auckland
Bogotá   Caracas   Lisbon   London   Madrid
Mexico City   Milan   Montreal   New Delhi
San Juan   Singapore   Sydney   Tokyo   Toronto

Preventive Medicine and Public Health: PreTest® Self-Assessment and Review

Copyright © 1995 1992 1989 1987 1985 1980 1976 by McGraw-Hill, Inc. All rights reserved. Printed in the United States of America. Except as permitted under the Copyright Act of 1976, no part of this publication may be reproduced or distributed in any form or by any means, or stored in a data base or retrieval system, without the prior written permission of the publisher.

1 2 3 4 5 6 7 8 9 0   DOCDOC   9 9 8 7 6 5 4

ISBN 0-07-052066-6

The editors were Gail Gavert and Bruce MacGregor.
The production supervisor was Gyl A. Favours.
R.R. Donnelley & Sons was printer and binder.
This book was set in Times Roman by Compset, Inc.

Library of Congress Cataloging-in-Publication Data

Preventive medicine and public health : Pretest® self-assessment and review.—
7th ed. / edited by F. Douglas Scutchfield.
   p. cm.
Includes bibliographical references.
ISBN 0-07-052066-6
   1. Public health—Examinations, questions, etc.   2. Medicine, Preventive—
Examinations, questions, etc.   3. Epidemiology—Examinations, questions, etc.   I. Scutchfield, F. Douglas.
RA430.E65   1994
362.1'076—dc20   93-38984

Contents

Preface

This is my first time editing this volume. I have tried to remain true, in the editing, to the intention of this book and hope you benefit from my efforts. I also hope you will realize, from review of this material, the importance of preventive medicine and public health to the contemporary practice of medicine. My discipline frequently suffers from a lack of recognition and respect in the medical curriculum. I believe that will not always be the case, but I have always been an optimist.

This book is dedicated to my parents, Ann and Beecher—"As the twig is bent, the tree's inclined"—and my students, who have taught me a great deal.

F. Douglas Scutchfield, M.D.

Introduction

Preventive Medicine and Public Health: PreTest® Self-Assessment and Review, 7/e, has been designed to provide medical students, as well as physicians, with a comprehensive and convenient instrument for self-assessment and review within the field of epidemiology and public health. The 500 questions provided have been designed to parallel the format of the questions contained in Step 2 of the United States Medical Licensing Examination (USMLE).

Each question in the book is accompanied by an answer, a paragraph explanation, and a specific page reference to either a current journal article, a textbook, or both. A bibliography that lists all the sources used in the book follows the last chapter.

Perhaps the most effective way to use this book is to allow yourself one minute to answer each question in a given chapter; as you proceed, indicate your answer beside each question. By following this suggestion, you will be approximating the time limits imposed by licensing examinations.

When you practice your examination-taking skills with this PreTest®, one way to maximize your score is to go through, answer all the questions you find easy, and skip over the more difficult ones initially. We do recommend, however, that once you come back to the more difficult questions, you spend as much time as you need to. You will then be more likely to retain the information. DO NOTE: When it comes to your examination for the board, you will do better to answer each question as you come to it and *not* skip around. Do not spend too much time on any one problem. Make a guess, circle the question, and come back to it. Otherwise, you can waste time looking on the computer score sheets for the question numbers you skipped or—the ultimate tragedy—you may discover that you forgot to skip a question and all your answers are off by one or more and time is running out.

When you have finished answering the questions in a chapter, you should then spend as much time as you need verifying your answers and carefully reading the explanations. Although you should pay special attention to the explanations for the questions you answered incorrectly, you should read every explanation. The author of this book has designed the explanations to reinforce and supplement the information tested by the questions. If, after reading the explanations for a given chapter, you feel you need still more information about the material covered, you may wish to consult the references indicated.

Biostatistics and Methods of Epidemiology

DIRECTIONS: Each question below contains five suggested responses. Select the **one best** response to each question.

1. Epidemiology can be defined as the study of

(A) the etiology of disease in humans
(B) the frequency of causes of death in humans
(C) the determinants of frequency of disease in humans
(D) the distribution and determinants of frequency of disease in humans
(E) the patterns of organization and financing of health care

2. A sample of 1000 people includes 120 who are hearing-impaired and 50 who are diabetic. If the number who are both diabetic and hearing-impaired is 6, then which of the following is true?

(A) Diabetes and hearing impairment appear to be independent characteristics
(B) Diabetics appear to be protected from hearing impairment
(C) Diabetics appear to be at greater risk of hearing impairment
(D) There is an interaction between diabetes and hearing impairment
(E) There is insufficient information to make any of the statements above

3. As an epidemiological investigation officer for the Centers for Disease Control and Prevention, you are contacted by a local health department. They inform you that a large number of persons have acquired mild symptoms of influenza despite being vaccinated for the appropriate strain being cultured. You find that the cultured strain is the same as that incorporated into the trivalent vaccine administered throughout the world. You also note that the strain had a high case fatality rate in previous epidemics in China, where most new strains are isolated and identified for vaccine preparations. The most likely explanation for the outbreak noted by the local health department is

(A) vaccine failure
(B) antigenic drift
(C) antigenic shift
(D) herd immunity
(E) incomplete immunity from previous rhinovirus infections

4. The association between low birth weight and maternal smoking during pregnancy can be studied by obtaining smoking histories from women at the time of the prenatal visit and then subsequently correlating birth weight with smoking histories. What type of study is this?

(A) Clinical trial
(B) Cross-sectional
(C) Cohort (prospective)
(D) Case-control (retrospective)
(E) None of the above

5. An investigator wishes to perform a randomized clinical trial to evaluate a new beta blocker as a treatment for hypertension. To be eligible for the study, subjects must have a resting diastolic blood pressure of at least 90 mmHg. One hundred patients seen at the screening clinic with this level of hypertension are recruited for the study and make appointments with the study nurse. When the nurse obtains their blood pressure 2 weeks later, only 65 of them have diastolic blood pressures of 90 mmHg or more. The most likely explanation for this is

(A) spontaneous resolution
(B) regression toward the mean
(C) baseline drift
(D) measurement error
(E) Hawthorne effect

6. All the following statements concerning the populations at risk for sexually transmitted disease (STD) are true EXCEPT

(A) there is an increased percentage of sexually experienced young persons
(B) the number of male homosexuals in proportion to other high-risk groups has increased
(C) baby-boomers have passed through the most sexually active and high-risk years
(D) continued high birth rates have increased the proportion of those with the highest rate for STD, low-income minority heterosexuals
(E) migration patterns and economic shifts have led to an increased concentration of low-income minorities in inner cities

7. Which of the following measures is used frequently as a denominator to calculate the incidence rate of a disease?

(A) Number of cases observed
(B) Number of new cases observed
(C) Number of asymptomatic cases
(D) Person-years of observation
(E) Persons lost to follow-up

8. A study is undertaken to determine whether use of Scutchfield's *PreTest Self-Assessment and Review* reduces sexual dysfunction related to anxiety before board examinations. One group of students studying for their board examinations was given the book to read; the other was not. The results are as follows:

Outcome	Got Book	Did Not Get Book
Sexual dysfunction	3	34
No sexual dysfunction	61	32

All the following statements are true EXCEPT

(A) these data could be analyzed using the chi-square test
(B) about half of the control group experienced sexual dysfunction
(C) unless one knows on what basis group assignment was made (i.e., randomized or not), the results are difficult to interpret
(D) the difference is probably due to chance
(E) a t test is inappropriate to analyze the data because the variables are categorical rather than continuous

9. Public health policies for the prevention and control of Lyme disease include all the following EXCEPT

(A) closure of endemic areas during peak infectious months
(B) notification of health providers concerning increased cases
(C) treatment of individuals with tetracycline for 10 to 30 days
(D) education of the public concerning self-protective measures
(E) control of intermediate hosts, such as deer and wild rodents

10. In 1971, the crude birth rate in the United States was approximately 17 per 1000 population; the death rate was 10 per 1000; and the net in-migration rate was 2 per 1000. What was the net growth rate per 1000?

(A) 5
(B) 7
(C) 9
(D) 15
(E) 25

11. In nine families surveyed, the numbers of children per family were 4, 6, 2, 2, 4, 3, 2, 1, and 7. The mean, median, and mode numbers of children per family are, respectively,

(A) 3.4, 2, 3
(B) 3, 3.4, 2
(C) 3, 3, 2
(D) 2, 3.5, 3
(E) none of the above

Questions 12–14

The results of a study of the incidence of pulmonary tuberculosis in a village in India are given in the table below. All persons in the village are examined during two surveys made 2 years apart, and the number of new cases was used to determine the incidence rate.

Category of Household at First Survey	Number of Persons	Number of New Cases
With culture-positive case	500	10
Without culture-positive case	10,000	10

12. What is the incidence of new cases per 1000 person-years in households that had a culture-positive case during the first survey?

(A) 0.02
(B) 0.01
(C) 1.0
(D) 10
(E) 20

13. What is the incidence of new cases per 1000 person-years in households that did not have a culture-positive case during the first survey?

(A) 0.001
(B) 0.1
(C) 0.5
(D) 1.0
(E) 5.0

14. What is the relative risk of acquiring tuberculosis in households with a culture-positive case compared with households without tuberculosis?

(A) 0.05
(B) 0.5
(C) 2.0
(D) 10
(E) 20

15. During the investigation of an outbreak of food poisoning at a summer camp, food histories were obtained from all campers as indicated in the table below. Which of the food items was probably responsible for the outbreak?

	Food	Proportion III (Percent)	
		Campers Who Ate Specified Food	Campers Who Did Not Eat Specified Food
(A)	Hamburger	61	48
(B)	Potatoes	70	35
(C)	Ice cream	40	50
(D)	Chicken	73	10
(E)	Lemonade	20	45

16. All the following statements concerning statistical inference are true EXCEPT

(A) a test of statistical significance does not prove causality

(B) a statistically significant test assesses the probability of a "chance" occurrence

(C) a statistically significant test supports the null hypothesis

(D) a confidence interval does not address whether an association is due to bias

(E) a confidence interval gives statistical significance as well as information concerning sample size

17. In the study of the cause of a disease, the essential difference between an *experimental* study and an *observational* study is that in the experimental investigation

(A) the study is prospective

(B) the study is retrospective

(C) the study and control groups are of equal size

(D) the study and control groups are selected on the basis of history of exposure to the suspected causal factor

(E) the investigators determine who is and who is not exposed to the suspected causal factor

Questions 18–19

About 1 percent of boys are born with undescended testes. To determine whether prenatal exposure to tobacco smoke is a cause of undescended testes in newborns, the mothers of 100 newborns with undescended testes and 100 newborns whose testes had descended were questioned about smoking habits during pregnancy. The study revealed an odds ratio of 2.6 associated with exposure to smoke, with 95 percent confidence intervals from 1.1 to 5.3.

18. Which of the following statements is true?

(A) The odds ratio could be falsely elevated by the inclusion of infants whose testes were descended (but retractile) in the case group (misclassification bias)

(B) The odds ratio would be falsely reduced if parents of affected infants were more likely to remember or report their smoking (recall bias)

(C) Because the cases are newborns, but the exposure data came from their mothers, this is not a true case-control study

(D) Since the study was not blinded, it is impossible to rule out a placebo effect

(E) None of the above

19. Which of the following statements is true?

(A) The results provide no evidence that maternal cigarette smoking is associated with undescended testes in the offspring

(B) If the study results are accurate, they suggest that a baby boy whose mother smoked is about 2.6 times as likely to be born with testes undescended as a baby boy whose mother did not smoke

(C) The fact that the confidence interval excludes 1.0 indicates that $p > 0.05$

(D) The 90 percent confidence interval for these results would probably include 1.0

(E) None of the above

20. The probability of being born with condition A is 0.10 and the probability of being born with condition B is 0.50. If conditions A and B are independent, what is the probability of being born with either condition A or condition B (or both)?

(A) 0.05
(B) 0.40
(C) 0.50
(D) 0.55
(E) 0.60

21. As an epidemiologist you are asked to recommend the type of study appropriate to the needs of researchers who would like to study the causes of a rare form of sarcoma. They have discovered a registry of this form of cancer and have access to a large data base of patients, which unfortunately is only a few years old. They have funding for only 1 year from the National Institutes of Health and note the budget will be tight. What type of study design do you recommend?

(A) Cohort (prospective)
(B) Historical cohort
(C) Cross-sectional
(D) Experimental
(E) Case-control (retrospective)

22. All the following are steps necessary to plan and conduct a care-control study EXCEPT

(A) developing and testing research instruments
(B) defining the disease and exposure of interest
(C) selecting cases and defining a control group
(D) planning the analysis
(E) determining the duration of the observational (study) period

23. All the following statements regarding the normal (Gaussian) distribution are true EXCEPT

(A) the mean = median = mode
(B) about 95 percent of observations fall within 2 standard deviations of the mean
(C) approximately 68 percent of observations fall within 1 standard deviation of the mean
(D) the number of observations between 0 and 1 standard deviation from the mean is the same as the number between 1 and 2 standard deviations from the mean
(E) the shape of the curve does not depend on the value of the mean

Questions 24–26

Lou Stewells, a pioneer in the study of diarrheal disease, has developed a new diagnostic test for cholera. When his agent is added to the stool, the organisms develop a characteristic ring around them. (He calls it the "Ring-Around-the-Cholera" [RAC] test.) He performs the test on 100 patients known to have cholera and 100 patients known not to have cholera with the following results:

	Cholera	No Cholera
RAC test +	91	12
RAC test −	9	88
Totals	100	100

24. All the following statements about the RAC test are correct EXCEPT

(A) the sensitivity of the test was about 91 percent
(B) the specificity of the test was about 12 percent
(C) the false negative rate was about 9 percent
(D) the predictive value of a positive result cannot be determined from the information above
(E) the predictive value of a negative result cannot be determined from the information above

25. Dr. Stewells next performs the test on 1000 patients with profuse diarrhea:

	Cholera	No Cholera
RAC test +	312	79
RAC test −	31	578
Totals	343	657

Which statement is correct?

(A) The predictive value of a positive result is 312/343
(B) The predictive value of a positive result is 79/312
(C) The predictive value of a negative result is 578/(578 + 31)
(D) The incidence rate of cholera in this population is 343/1000
(E) None of the above

26. The RAC test achieves widespread acceptance. However, with improvements in hygiene, the prevalence of cholera gradually falls from 35 to 5 percent of hospitalized diarrhea patients. Which statement about the effect of this fall in prevalence is true?

(A) The change in prevalence will reduce the predictive value of a negative result
(B) The predictive value of a positive result will decline
(C) The specificity of the test is likely to decline
(D) The specificity of the test will increase at the expense of its sensitivity
(E) None of the above

27. Randomization is a procedure used for assignment or allocation of subjects to treatment and control groups in experimental studies. Randomization ensures

(A) that assignment occurs by chance
(B) that treatment and control groups are alike in all respects except treatment
(C) that bias in observations is eliminated
(D) that placebo effects are eliminated
(E) none of the above

28. In comparing the difference between two means, the value of p is found to be 0.60. The correct interpretation of this result is

(A) the null hypothesis is rejected
(B) the difference is compatible with the null hypothesis
(C) the difference occurred by chance
(D) the difference is statistically significant
(E) sampling variation is an unlikely explanation of the difference

29. In a study of the cause of lung cancer, patients who had the disease were matched with controls by age, sex, place of residence, and social class. The frequency of cigarette smoking was then compared in the two groups. What type of study was this?

(A) Cohort (prospective)
(B) Historical cohort
(C) Clinical trial
(D) Case-control (retrospective)
(E) None of the above

30. As a new public health officer, you are tasked with developing criteria for a disease surveillance system. All the following are important purposes for a public health surveillance system EXCEPT

(A) detection of epidemics
(B) detection of rare but fatal conditions, such as Alzheimer's disease
(C) description of trends and the natural history of a health condition
(D) evaluation of hypotheses about the occurrence of a disease
(E) evaluation of control and prevention measures

Questions 31–33

Smoking and alcohol use are both risk factors for esophageal cancer. The hypothetical table below shows how the incidence of esophageal cancer varies with either smoking or alcohol use (but not both):

| | Incidence (cases/10,000 person-yr) | |
	Nonsmoker	Smoker
Nondrinker	10	50
Drinker	30	X

31. All the following statements are true EXCEPT

(A) in nonsmokers, the excess risk of esophageal cancer from drinking is 20 cases per 10,000 person-years
(B) in nondrinkers, the relative risk of esophageal cancer from smoking is 5.0
(C) the overall relative risk for smoking cannot be determined without knowledge of X and the proportion of the population that drinks
(D) the table shows that smoking causes more cases of esophageal cancer in this population than does drinking
(E) in nondrinkers, the excess risk of esophageal cancer from smoking is 40 cases per 10,000 person-years.

32. If smoking and alcohol act independently to cause esophageal cancer under an *additive* model, what would be the expected value of X?

(A) 60
(B) 70
(C) 80
(D) 150
(E) None of the above

33. If smoking and alcohol act independently according to a *multiplicative* model, what would be the expected value of X?

(A) 70
(B) 80
(C) 120
(D) 1500
(E) None of the above

34. In the table below, data are presented on the number of children suffering from acute leukemia who were admitted to a hospital between 1970 and 1984. Correct conclusions about the data include which of the following?

| Age (years) | Number of Children Admitted in Interval | | |
	1970–74	1975–79	1980–84
0–4	12	23	31
5–9	8	17	36
10–14	10	7	4
Total	30	47	71

(A) The incidence rate of leukemia decreased in children 10 to 14 years old
(B) The prevalence rate of leukemia increased in children between 1970 and 1984
(C) The incidence rate of leukemia increased in children 5 to 9 years old
(D) The number of children 9 years old and under admitted to the study hospital because of acute leukemia increased between 1970 and 1984
(E) None of the above

35. The Coronary Drug Project was a randomized trial to evaluate the efficacy of several lipid-lowering drugs. The 5-year mortality of the men who adhered to the regimen of clofibrate (i.e., took 80 percent of their medicine or more) was 15 percent; among those assigned to the clofibrate group who were less compliant, it was 24.6 percent. The result was highly statistically significant ($p = 0.0001$). From this one can conclude

(A) clofibrate was very beneficial to the patients who took it reliably
(B) clofibrate is not effective unless patients take at least 80 percent of the recommended doses
(C) either clofibrate or something associated with taking it reliably is strongly associated with reduced total mortality
(D) there was a problem with blinding in this study
(E) none of the above

36. The prevalence of smoking in a certain population is 25 percent. The lung cancer rate for smokers is 125/100,000. The lung cancer rate for nonsmokers is 5/100,000. The case fatality rate for smokers and nonsmokers is equal. What is the percentage of deaths from lung cancer that can be attributed to smoking?

(A) 31 percent
(B) 55 percent
(C) 80 percent
(D) 96 percent
(E) None of the above

37. A randomized, double-blinded trial finds that oral corticosteroids are superior to placebo in hastening the resolution of otitis media with effusion. Possible reasons why this study might have given a falsely positive result include

(A) the sample size may have been too small
(B) the apparent effect might be a result of chance
(C) it may be difficult to determine accurately which effusions have resolved, which will lead to errors in determining the outcome of the study
(D) lax inclusion criteria may have led to inclusion of some subjects in the study who did not really have otitis media with effusion
(E) none of the above

38. Which of the following results gives the reader the most information concerning statistical significance, sample size, and strength of association?

(A) A relative risk of 2.5 with a 95 percent confidence interval of 2.0 to 3.1
(B) A p value of 0.0004 and an alpha $(\alpha) = 0.05$
(C) A relative risk of 5.0 with a 95 percent confidence interval of 0.1 to 9.8
(D) A p value of <0.05 and a relative risk of 2.5
(E) A relative risk of 5.0 and a statistical power of 0.70

39. An investigator is designing a randomized clinical trial to see whether vitamin E will prevent cancer in smokers. Which of the following is the LEAST important consideration in planning the sample size for the study?

(A) The expected incidence of cancer in the placebo group
(B) The frequency with which subjects are likely to be lost to follow-up or die from non-cancer causes over the duration of the study
(C) The prevalence of smoking in the population
(D) The values for alpha and beta, the type 1 and type 2 error rates
(E) The magnitude of the preventive effect that the investigator wishes to be able to detect

40. During an epidemiological investigation, which of the following steps would most likely follow comparison of the hypothesis with the established facts?

(A) Determination of who is at risk of having the health problem
(B) Confirmation of the diagnosis
(C) Estimation of the number of cases
(D) Orientation of the data in terms of time, place, and person
(E) Proposal of measures for control and prevention

41. All the following are advantages of case-control studies, as opposed to cohort studies, EXCEPT

(A) they are relatively quick studies
(B) they allow calculation of exposure rates
(C) they can study many possible causes of a disease
(D) they require relatively few study subjects
(E) they can easily study rare diseases

42. In a case-control study to determine the association between blood type and invasive cervical cancer, the authors examined the distribution of ABO blood type among those with cervical cancer and matched controls without cervical cancer. The authors chose male subjects for controls, which were matched to cases as female subjects would be. Which one of the following statements about the study design is correct?

(A) Because males cannot get cervical cancer, recall bias would be eliminated in the study
(B) Inclusion of males would increase the difficulty of finding matched controls
(C) Inclusion of males would tend to overestimate the risk of cervical cancer
(D) The distribution of ABO blood type is not sex-dependent and thus would be the same for matched controls of either sex
(E) None of the above

43. The crude death rate in the United States is 150/100,000. The crude death rate in a smaller, developing country is 75/100,000. Based on these data, which one of the following statements is correct?

(A) The health care system of the developing country is far better than that in the United States

(B) More people die in the United States because it has a larger population

(C) Infant mortality in the first week is higher in developing countries, but it is not included in the crude death rate

(D) Death rates in the developing country are lower due to the emigration effect

(E) Crude death rates are usually higher in developed countries because of a higher proportion of older persons in the population

44. True statements concerning cohort studies include all the following EXCEPT

(A) cohort studies are longitudinal in design

(B) subjects are selected on the basis of characteristics present before the onset of the condition being studied

(C) subjects are observed over time to determine the frequency of occurrence of the condition under study

(D) cohort studies can be retrospective

(E) cohort studies are necessary to estimate the prevalence of diseases

Questions 45–48

A research team wishes to investigate a possible association between smokeless tobacco and oral lesions among professional baseball players. At spring training camp, they ask each baseball player about current and past use of smokeless tobacco, cigarettes, and alcohol, and a dentist notes the type and extent of the lesions in the mouth.

45. What type of study is this?

(A) Case-control
(B) Cross-sectional
(C) Cohort
(D) Clinical trial
(E) None of the above

46. After the players have been questioned about use of smokeless tobacco and examined for lesions of the mouth, the data on the 146 players are tabulated as follows:

	Mouth Lesion	No Lesion	Total
User	80	30	110
Non-user	2	34	36
Total	82	64	146

In this study, what is the incidence rate of mouth lesions among the baseball players who use smokeless tobacco?

(A) 80/30
(B) 80/110
(C) 82/146
(D) 30/110
(E) Cannot be calculated from the data given

47. All the following statements about the association between use of smokeless tobacco and oral lesions in this study are true EXCEPT

(A) the odds ratio is (80 × 34)/(2 × 30) = 45.3
(B) users of smokeless tobacco are about 45.3 times as likely as nonusers to have oral lesions
(C) the prevalence of use of smokeless tobacco in this sample is 110/146
(D) the results are likely to be statistically significant
(E) the statistical significance could be calculated using a chi-square test

48. If the association between use of smokeless tobacco and oral lesions in the last question is causal, approximately what proportion of the mouth lesions in the smokers is due to use of smokeless tobacco?

(A) 27 percent
(B) 50 percent
(C) 73 percent
(D) 92 percent
(E) 99 percent

49. For many diagnostic or screening tests, there is a tradeoff between sensitivity and specificity. True statements include which of the following?

(A) Sensitivity would be extremely important when testing for amyotrophic lateral sclerosis (ALS) because there is no good treatment for it

(B) Because hypothyroidism in infancy is devastating if missed, a screening test for it should be highly specific

(C) Specificity is more important than sensitivity for screening tests

(D) In evaluating the potential usefulness of a screening test, the effectiveness of treatment for the disease screened for is important

(E) None of the above

50. The occurrence of a group of illnesses of similar nature at a rate above the expected number is called

(A) hyperendemic
(B) epidemic
(C) endemic
(D) enzootic
(E) pandemic

51. The time interval between entry of an infectious agent into a host and the onset of symptoms is called

(A) the communicable period
(B) the incubation period
(C) the preinfectious period
(D) the noncontagious period
(E) the decubation period

52. A randomized trial shows that a new thrombolytic agent reduces total mortality in the first 30 days after a suspected myocardial infarction by 30 percent compared with a placebo ($p < 0.002$). Which of the following questions would be the most important to have answered?

(A) Was the trial blinded?
(B) What was the power of the study?
(C) What happened to surviving patients in the next year?
(D) What percentage of patients in each group actually had a myocardial infarction?
(E) What was the effect on mortality from coronary heart disease?

53. A radiologist develops a new screening test for cancer of the pancreas. The sensitivity and specificity of the test are said to be "very high, at least 98 percent." You are asked to determine whether it would be useful to screen everyone in your primary care practice with this test in the next year. To answer, you would need to know all the following EXCEPT

(A) the incidence of asymptomatic pancreatic cancer
(B) the prevalence of asymptomatic pancreatic cancer
(C) the exact values of the sensitivity and specificity of the tests
(D) the cost of the test
(E) the survival rate from pancreatic cancer cases detected by the new test

Questions 54–56

In a study of the effectiveness of pertussis vaccine in preventing pertussis (whooping cough), the following data were collected by studying siblings of children who had the disease.

Immunization Status of Sibling Contact	Number of Siblings Exposed to Case	Number of Cases among Siblings
Complete	4000	400
None	1000	400

54. What was the secondary attack rate of pertussis in fully immunized household contacts?

(A) 0 percent
(B) 10 percent
(C) 25 percent
(D) 40 percent
(E) 75 percent

55. What was the protective efficacy of whooping cough vaccine?

(A) 25 percent
(B) 40 percent
(C) 75 percent
(D) 90 percent
(E) None of the above

56. What was the relative risk of contracting whooping cough in the unimmunized children compared with the fully immunized children?

(A) 0.25
(B) 0.5
(C) 1.0
(D) 2.0
(E) 4.0

Questions 57–59

Data from an investigation of an epidemic of German measles in a remote village in Brazil are given in the table below:

Age Group (years)	Number in Population	Number Ill (symptomatic)	Number Not Ill but with Antibody Rise (asymptomatic)	Number Uninfected	Percent Infected
0–9	204	110	74	20	90
10–19	129	70	46	13	90
20–39	161	88	57	16	90
40–59	78	42	28	8	90
60+	42	2	2	38	10
Totals	614	312	207	95	

57. Which expression represents the calculation to determine the incidence of illness for all age groups (as a percentage)?

(A) $\dfrac{95}{519} \times 100\% = 18.3\%$

(B) $\dfrac{207}{614} \times 100\% = 33.7\%$

(C) $\dfrac{207}{519} \times 100\% = 39.9\%$

(D) $\dfrac{312}{614} \times 100\% = 50.8\%$

(E) $\dfrac{519}{614} \times 100\% = 84.5\%$

58. Which expression represents the calculation to determine the percentage of infection that is asymptomatic (subclinical)?

(A) $\dfrac{95}{519} \times 100\% = 18.3\%$

(B) $\dfrac{207}{614} \times 100\% = 33.7\%$

(C) $\dfrac{207}{519} \times 100\% = 39.9\%$

(D) $\dfrac{312}{614} \times 100\% = 50.8\%$

(E) $\dfrac{519}{614} \times 100\% = 84.5\%$

59. Based on the age-specific infection rates, when did German measles previously occur in this village—in relation to the current epidemic?

(A) 1 to 9 years ago
(B) 10 to 19 years ago
(C) 20 to 39 years ago
(D) 40 to 59 years ago
(E) 60 years ago

60. The authors of a study state that careful autopsies show that 60 percent of all persons who die have evidence of recent or previous pulmonary embolism and conclude that pulmonary embolism is the leading cause of death in the U.S. Possible reasons for disagreeing with the conclusion include all the following EXCEPT

(A) confounding
(B) selection bias
(C) random error
(D) lack of definition of pulmonary embolism
(E) lead-time bias

61. "The absence of valvular calcification in an adult suggests that severe valvular aortic stenosis is not present." This statement means that

(A) valvular calcification is a sensitive test for severe valvular aortic stenosis
(B) valvular calcification is an insensitive test for severe valvular aortic stenosis
(C) valvular calcification is a specific test for severe valvular aortic stenosis
(D) valvular calcification is a nonspecific test for severe valvular aortic stenosis
(E) the positive predictive value of valvular calcification is high

62. The primary way to increase precision of a study is to increase the sample size. Sample size can be calculated given certain study parameters. All the following parameters are used to calculate sample size EXCEPT

(A) level of statistical significance (α error)
(B) the null hypothesis (H_0)
(C) magnitude of effect
(D) chance of missing a real effect (β error)
(E) ratio of cases to controls

63. In a previously well 35-year-old man with 3 h of severe, crushing substernal chest pain and 5 mm of acute ST elevation in leads V_2 to V_4 application of Bayesian reasoning would indicate that

(A) he is likely to have a nonatherosclerotic form of coronary heart disease
(B) he is likely to have a serum cholesterol above 9 mmol/L (326 mg/dL)
(C) he is likely to be having an acute myocardial infarction
(D) an elevated level of a creatine kinase MB isozyme is likely to be a false positive
(E) measurement of creatine kinase MB isozymes would not be a very sensitive test

64. Decision analyses often include a patient's utilities in the determination of the best decision. These utilities measure

(A) whether a patient favors one decision over another
(B) whether a physician favors one decision over another
(C) the difference between a patient's decision and the physician's decision
(D) the relative value a patient places on a particular outcome
(E) the relative likelihood of a particular outcome

65. All the following statements concerning meta-analysis are true EXCEPT

(A) it is a study in which the units of analysis are populations or groups of people, rather than individuals
(B) it is used to enhance the statistical power of research findings where numbers in available studies are too small
(C) it is applied by pooling results of small, randomized, controlled trials when no single trial has large enough numbers to reach statistical significance
(D) it combines results from different studies to obtain a numerical estimate of an overall effect
(E) it is meant to be more objective and quantitative than a narrative review

66. Studies in medicine are designed to identify causes of disease. The ultimate goal of such studies is to alter the frequency or severity of these diseases. All the following are considerations in the determination of causality EXCEPT

(A) temporal sequence—causative agents must precede their consequences
(B) biological gradient—dose-response curve
(C) concurrency—cause and effect are found at the same time
(D) strength of association
(E) consistency—repeated observations of the same associations

DIRECTIONS: Each group of questions below consists of lettered headings followed by a set of numbered items. For each numbered item select the **one** lettered heading with which it is **most** closely associated. Each lettered heading may be used **once, more than once, or not at all.**

Questions 67–70

For each of the studies below, choose the most appropriate statistical test to analyze the data.

(A) Chi-square analysis
(B) Student t test
(C) Paired t test
(D) Analysis of variance
(E) Linear regression

67. Comparison of systolic blood pressures in independent samples of pregnant and nonpregnant women

68. Comparison of the prevalence of hepatitis B surface antigen (HBsAg) in medical and dental students

69. Comparison of the level of blood glucose in male and female rats following administration of three different drugs

70. Comparison of serum cholesterol before and after ingestion of hamburgers in a sample of fast-food patrons

Questions 71–74

For each of the following descriptions, pick the appropriate epidemiologic term.

(A) Confounding
(B) Effect modification (interaction)
(C) Misclassification bias
(D) Lead-time bias
(E) None of the above

71. Elevated bilirubin levels in neonates are associated with brain damage only in babies who also have infections or severe hemolytic disease

72. People who drink coffee tend to smoke more, and for this reason coffee drinkers have a higher risk of lung cancer

73. Higher lead levels in hyperactive children may be due to increased consumption of paint in children who were already hyperactive

74. The association between blood lead levels and IQ may be a result of the fact that both are associated with socioeconomic status

Questions 75–78

In each statement below, data are presented based on a cohort study of coronary heart disease. Choose the parameter that best describes each of these statements.

(A) Point prevalence
(B) Incidence rate
(C) Standardized morbidity ratio
(D) Relative risk
(E) None of the above

75. At the initial examination, 17 persons per 1000 had evidence of coronary heart disease (CHD)

76. Among heavy smokers, the observed frequency of angina pectoris was 1.6 times as great as the expected frequency during the first 12 years of the study

77. During the first 8 years of the study, 45 persons developed coronary heart disease per 1000 persons who entered the study free of disease

78. The risk of coronary heart disease was 23 percent higher in relatives of patients with CHD than in the general population

Questions 79–83

Match the examples below with the appropriate epidemiologic terms.

(A) Lead-time bias
(B) Surveillance bias
(C) Recall bias
(D) Type 1 error
(E) Power

79. Medical students who fail a physiology examination are more likely to report missing two or more physiology lectures than those who fail a neuroanatomy examination

80. The chance of discovering the truth that twice as many of your friends are at the movies as are studying for their board examinations

81. In a class of 150 medical students, there will likely be a few who can answer this question correctly without understanding the material

82. The likelihood of finding a lost biochemistry notebook in your apartment is higher in the month of June than in the month of March

83. Medical students enrolled in a first-year anatomy class are more likely to remain at their same addresses for the next 2 years than medical students enrolled in fourth-year clerkships

Questions 84–87

Choose the rate that best describes each statement below.

(A) Secondary attack rate
(B) Case fatality rate
(C) Morbidity rate
(D) Age-adjusted mortality
(E) Crude mortality

84. Death occurs in 10 percent of cases of meningococcal meningitis

85. Approximately 9 people die each year in the United States for every 1000 estimated to be alive

86. Eighty percent of susceptible household contacts of a child with chickenpox develop this disease

87. Children between the ages of 1 and 5 have an average of eight colds per year

Questions 88–91

Choose the term that best fits the description.

(A) Matching
(B) Stratification
(C) Age adjustment
(D) Multivariate statistical analysis
(E) Survival analysis

88. In a cohort study of hypertensive men, the proportions of subjects with high and low renin levels who survived for 5 years are compared separately among those aged 40 to 49, those aged 50 to 59, and those aged 60 to 69 at entry

89. A sampling strategy is used to achieve comparability of the groups being studied

90. A technique that takes into account variable length of follow-up is used

91. Six different risk ratios are calculated: one for each sex at each of three social class levels

Questions 92–95

For each of the studies described below, select the critical statement that best explains why the conclusion is misleading or false.

(A) Lack of a control group
(B) Lack of proper follow-up
(C) Lack of adjustment for age
(D) Lack of denominators
(E) Lack of adjustment for race

92. Of 250 consecutive, unselected women in whom acute cholecystitis was diagnosed, 75 were under age 50 and 175 were over age 50. The investigator concluded that older women are at greater risk of acute cholecystitis than are younger women.

93. In a review of 3000 patients in whom adult-onset diabetes was diagnosed, 2000 of these patients were obese at the time of diagnosis. The investigator concluded that there is an association between diabetes and obesity

94. Acute anxiety neurosis was diagnosed among 250 patients and follow-up data were available on 80 percent of these patients 10 years later. The mortality experience of this cohort was no different from that of the general population. The authors concluded that the diagnosis of acute anxiety neurosis is not associated with a decrease in longevity

95. Of 143 patients who died of bacterial endocarditis and on whom autopsies were performed, 2 percent were less than 10 years of age. The authors concluded that bacterial endocarditis is rare in childhood

Questions 96–99

For each of the descriptions of statistical procedures below, choose the statistical error.

(A) Observations are not independent
(B) Variable is not normally distributed
(C) Unequal group sizes or unequal variances exist
(D) Degrees of freedom are insufficient
(E) None of the above

96. The frequencies of infection of the urinary tract are compared in 24 children treated with intermittent catheterization and 9 children treated with urinary diversion. In the catheterization group, 85/231 urine cultures were positive, compared with 34/55 in the diversion group. The difference between these two proportions was statistically significant ($\chi^2 = 11.4$ degrees of freedom = 1.0, $p < 0.001$)

97. The mean lengths of hospital stay were compared in 20 premature infants treated surgically and 20 premature infants treated medically for patent ductus arteriosus. The mean lengths of stay in the two groups were 50 ± 30 and 30 ± 30 days (mean $\pm$ standard deviation), respectively. The test was not significant ($t = 1.5$, $p = 0.07$)

98. The parity of 100 women with breast cancer was compared with that of 200 controls. Among the cases, 40 percent were nulliparous, 30 percent had one child, and 30 percent had more than one child; among the controls the numbers were 20, 30, and 50 percent, respectively. The mean ($\pm$ SD) parity in the cases was 1.6 ± 2.1; in the controls it was 2.2 ± 2.3. The difference was statistically significant using the t test ($t = -2.2$; $p = 0.04$)

99. An investigator wishes to examine the efficacy of varicella vaccine. For convenience, he randomizes four classes of third graders for the study: two classes receive the vaccine and two do not. Over the next year, only 2/57 children in the vaccine group, but 25/60 children in the control group get chicken pox ($\chi^2 = 23$, degrees of freedom = 1.0, $p < 0.001$). The investigator concludes that the vaccine is highly effective.

Questions 100–103

The following two-by-two table represents the findings of a 5-year cohort study in which the incidence of suicide in veterans who served in Vietnam was compared with that of veterans who served elsewhere. Match the name of the parameter below with the appropriate formula.

	Suicide	No Suicide
Served in Vietnam	a	b
Served elsewhere	c	d

(A) ad/bc
(B) $(a + b)/(a + b + c + d)$
(C) $(a + c)/(a + b + c + d)$
(D) $[a/(a + b)]/[c/(c + d)]$
(E) $a/(a + b) - c/(c + d)$

100. The odds ratio

101. The relative risk

102. The excess risk of suicide in Vietnam veterans

103. The overall incidence (per 5 years) of suicide in the study)

Questions 104–107

Match each description of a sampling procedure with the correct term.

(A) Systematic sampling
(B) Paired sampling
(C) Simple random sampling
(D) Stratified sampling
(E) Cluster sampling

104. Each individual of the total group has an equal chance of being selected

105. Households are selected at random, and every person in each household is included in the sample

106. Individuals are initially assembled according to some order in a group and then individuals are selected according to some constant determinant; e.g., every fourth subject is selected

107. Individuals are divided into subgroups on the basis of specified characteristics and then random samples are selected from each subgroup

Questions 108–112

A new test for chlamydial infections of the cervix is introduced. Half of the women who are tested have a positive test. Compared with the gold standard of careful cultures, 45 percent of those with a positive test are infected with chlamydia, and 95 percent of those with a negative test are free of the infection. Match the epidemiologic terms below with the correct percentage.

(A) 5 percent
(B) 25 percent
(C) 80 percent
(D) 90 percent
(E) None of the above

108. Sensitivity of the test

109. Specificity of the test

110. Prevalence of chlamydial infection in that community

111. Predictive value of a positive test

112. Predictive value of a negative test

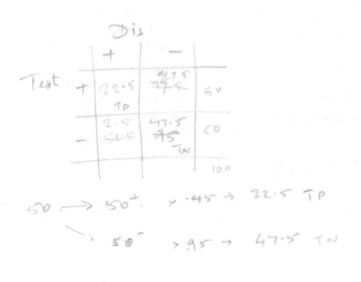

Questions 113–116

Select the letter corresponding to the figure that best fits each description.

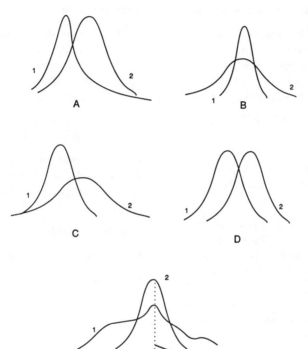

113. Distributions 1 and 2 have the same median and mean, but 2 has the greater variance

114. Distributions 1 and 2 have the same variance, but different means

115. Compared with curve 2, curve 1 is skewed to the right

116. This figure represents a tasty dessert

Questions 117–120

For each result or conclusion described below, select the choice that might best explain it.

(A) Ecologic fallacy
(B) Type 1 error
(C) Type 2 error
(D) Selection bias
(E) Misclassification bias

117. A randomized blinded trial of aspirin to prevent myocardial infarction fails to find a difference between aspirin and placebo groups after 5 years ($N = 500$ per group; $p = 0.11$)

118. A study of patterns of contraceptive use finds that counties with the highest per capita use of condoms also have the highest pregnancy rates ($N = 100,000$; $p < 0.001$) and concludes that condoms are ineffective as contraceptives

119. An investigator analyzes data from the National Health Interview Survey and finds that there is a positive association between consumption of turkey and degenerative joint disease in black women 50 to 59 years old ($N = 50$; $p < 0.05$)

120. In a case-control study of lung cancer, cases' spouses are chosen as controls. The odds ratio for smoking is 3.0, which does not quite reach statistical significance ($N = 30$ per group; $p = 0.07$)

Questions 121–125

For each variable described below, choose the type of measurement scale.

(A) Dichotomous scale
(B) Nominal scale
(C) Ordinal scale
(D) Interval scale
(E) Ratio scale

121. Survival of a particular patient for at least 5 years

122. Frequency of somnolence during biochemistry lectures: never, sometimes, usually, or always

123. Birth weight

124. Type of medical specialty

125. Year of birth

Questions 126–130

Dr. Vera Blues, a noted psychiatric epidemiologist, is interested in the diagnosis of depression. She develops a new test for its diagnosis, which she calls the Blues test. According to the gold standard, which involves meeting the *DSM-IV* criteria, about 1 percent of adults in the U.S. are depressed. Dr. Blues applies her new test to 100 persons diagnosed as being depressed by the gold standard; 80 have a positive Blues test. She finds 400 persons who are not depressed; again, 80 have a positive test. She reports her findings in the *Journal of the Society of Academic Psychiatrists (JSAP)*. Match the statements that Dr. Blues made in her article with the appropriate percentage.

(A) 80 percent
(B) 50 percent
(C) 20 percent
(D) < 1 percent
(E) None of the above

126. "I found that the sensitivity of the Blues test was . . ."

127. "The specificity of the Blues test was . . ."

128. "The likelihood that someone with depression would have a positive Blues test was . . ."

129. "The likelihood that someone in the population with a positive Blues test would be depressed was . . ."

130. "The likelihood that someone in the population with a negative Blues test would be depressed was . . ."

Biostatistics and Methods
of Epidemiology
Answers

1. The answer is D. *(Mausner, 2/e, p 1.)* The word *epidemiology* comes from the Greek words *epi* (upon) and *demos* (people). In fact, there is a separate word for the study of determinants of disease in animals—*epizootiology*. Epidemiology is the study of both the distribution of diseases in human populations and the determinants of the observed distribution. It began as the study of infectious diseases but has expanded to include the study of chronic diseases, organization of health care, delivery of health care, and occupational and environmental health.

2. The answer is A. *(Ingelfinger, 2/e, pp 11–12.)* Two characteristics are independent of each other (i.e., unrelated) if and only if the probability of both occurring in the same person is equal to the product of their probabilities. In this example, we estimate the probability of hearing impairment in this population as $120/1000 = 0.12$, and the probability of diabetes as $50/1000 = 0.05$. The product of these probabilities is $(0.12)(0.05) = 0.006$. Thus, with a sample size of 1000, if hearing impairment and diabetes were independent, we would expect about 6 persons to be both hearing-impaired and diabetic—exactly what was found.

3. The answer is B. *(Benenson, 15/e, pp 224–229. Last, Dictionary, 2/e, p 6.)* Antigenic drift is most likely the cause of changes in the strain that allowed infection despite adequate vaccination. Partial immunity or mutation to a less virulent strain (also due to antigenic drift) could be responsible for the less severe symptoms noted in this outbreak. Antigenic drift is a slow and progressive change in the antigenic composition of microorganisms. This alters the immunological responses of individuals and a population's susceptibility to that microorganism. Antigenic *shift* is a sudden change in the molecular structure of a microorganism and produces new strains. This results in little or no acquired immunity to these new strains and is the explanation for new epidemics or pandemics. Vaccine failure would result in influenza cases with high case fatality rates seen previously with this strain. Herd immunity would decrease the rate of infection by decreasing the probability that a susceptible person would come into contact with an infected person. This would not affect the clinical presentation of those infected. Influenza is not a rhinovirus and there is no cross-immunity between the two.

4. The answer is C. *(Mausner, 2/e, pp 156–158.)* This study is a *cohort* (prospective) study because the subjects (pregnant women) were categorized on the basis of exposure or lack of exposure to a risk factor (smoking during pregnancy), and then were followed to determine if a particular outcome (low-birth-weight babies) resulted. The term *cohort* refers to the group of subjects who are followed forward in time to see which ones develop the outcome. *Clinical trials* are prospective studies in which an *intervention* is applied—no intervention was mentioned in the question. In a *case-control* (retrospective) study of the relationship between low birth weight and maternal smoking, infants would be selected on the basis of low birth weight (cases) and normal birth weight (controls) and then the frequency of maternal smoking would be compared in the two groups. In *cross-sectional* studies exposure and outcome are measured at the same point in time.

5. The answer is B. *(Ingelfinger, 2/e, pp 189–191.)* Although hypertension can resolve spontaneously, this is an unlikely explanation for resolution over a 2-week period in 35 percent of the subjects. A much more likely explanation is *regression* toward the mean. Because of random fluctuations, any one measurement of blood pressure may be far from a person's normal blood pressure. By referring patients for the study based on a single measurement, those in whom the measurement was falsely high are much more likely to be referred than those in whom the measurement was too low. Thus in any group selected based on a characteristic with substantial day-to-day variation, many will have values closer to the population mean when the measurement is repeated. Neither baseline drift (which occurs with measurements on certain machines that require frequent calibration) nor measurement error is as likely an explanation. The Hawthorne effect refers to a tendency among study subjects to change simply because they are being studied. It is much more likely to affect studies of behavior or attitudes than a study of blood pressure.

6. The answer is B. *(Last, Maxcy-Rosenau, 13/e, p 100.)* The number of male homosexuals in proportion to other risk groups has not changed appreciably. However, the numbers of those sexually active and the proportion of those at highest risk have grown. Behavioral changes have significantly decreased STD rates among white male homosexuals, but this effect may be limited to the cohort targeted for education. Subsequent cohorts may return to the previously higher rates for STDs without continued educational intervention.

7. The answer is D. *(Mausner, 2/e, pp 46–48.)* Person-years of observation are frequently used in the denominator of incidence rates and provide a method of dealing with variable follow-up periods. Person-years of observation simultaneously take into account the number of persons under observation and the duration of observation of each person. For example, if 8 new cases of diabetes occurred among 1000 people followed for 2 years, the incidence would be 8 cases per 2000 person-years, or 4 per 1000 person-years of follow-up. The distinction between *rates* and *proportions* is not well maintained in standard epidemiologic terminology. Rates should have units of inverse time and will vary depending on the units of measurement of time; they can vary from 0 to infinity. However, such terms as *case fatality rate, attack rate,* and *prevalence rate* are in widespread usage even though technically they are all proportions; i.e., they vary between 0 and 1 and are unitless.

8. The answer is D. *(Colton, pp 129, 174.)* The data presented are for a dichotomous predictor variable (book/no book) and a dichotomous outcome variable (dysfunction/no dysfunction), so a chi-square test (but not a t test) is appropriate for analysis. Since there is apparently such a big difference between the groups, chance is not a likely explanation for the findings. It is essential to know how the groups were assigned if the study is to be properly interpreted. In fact, in this case, the control group was chosen from subjects at a clinic for sexual dysfunction.

9. The answer is C. *(Benenson, 15/e, pp 255–257. Last, Dictionary, 2/e, pp 14–29.)* Public education, surveillance systems, environmental control, and dissemination of information to health providers are all methods used in public health. Treatment of individuals with a few exceptions is traditionally left to individual practitioners. Generally, public health is concerned with population and group health as opposed to individual health.

10. The answer is C. *(Mausner, 2/e, pp 256–257.)* Net growth rate equals the birth rate minus the death rate plus the in-migration rate minus the out-migration rate: $(17 - 10) + 2 = 9$. Rates can be added or subtracted directly only if they are based on the same population denominator (in this case, the estimated midyear population).

11. The answer is E. *(Colton, pp 28–31.)* The correct values for mean, median, and mode are 3.4, 3, and 2. The *mean* is the average: the sum of the observations divided by the number of observations. In this case, the mean is $31 \div 9 = 3.4$. The *median* is the middle observation in a series of ordered observations, i.e., the 50th percentile (when the number of observations is even, it is midway between the two middle observations). In this case, when the observations are ordered—1, 2, 2, 2, 3, 4, 4, 6, 7—the median is 3. The *mode* is the observation that occurs with greatest frequency; in this case it is 2, which occurs three times.

12. The answer is D. *(Mausner, 2/e, pp 44–49.)* According to the table, 10 new cases of tuberculosis developed among the 500 persons belonging to households with a case of tuberculosis at the time of the first survey. Because these 500 persons were followed for 2 years, the number of person-years of exposure is 1000. Therefore, the incidence rate is calculated as follows:

$$\frac{10 \text{ new cases}}{500 \text{ persons} \times 2 \text{ years}} = 10 \text{ cases per 1000 person-years}$$

(See also question 8.)

13. The answer is C. *(Mausner, 2/e, pp 44–49.)* Ten new cases of tuberculosis developed among 10,000 persons belonging to households that had no culture-positive cases at the time of the first survey. Since these 10,000 persons were followed for 2 years, the number of person-years of exposure is 20,000. Therefore, the incidence rate is calculated as follows:

$$\frac{10 \text{ new cases}}{10,000 \text{ persons} \times 2 \text{ years}} = 0.5 \text{ cases per 1000 person-years}$$

14. The answer is E. *(Mausner, 2/e, p 169.)* The relative risk is the *ratio* of the incidence of a disease in a group exposed to a factor (in this case, household contact with tuberculosis) to the incidence in a group not exposed to the factor (persons without household contact). Therefore, the reactive risk is

$$\frac{\text{Incidence in households with exposure}}{\text{Incidence in households without exposure}} = \frac{10}{0.5} = 20$$

Identification of groups with a high level of relative risk can be useful in planning disease control programs.

15. The answer is D. *(Mausner, 2/e, pp 289–292.)* The identification of a specific factor (food) as a cause of illness (food poisoning) depends on comparing the proportion who become ill among those who did and those who did not eat each specified food (the proportion ill is sometimes called the "attack rate," but in fact it is a proportion, not a rate [see question 8]). The proportion ill among those who ate the food suspected of causing the disease should be significantly greater than among those who did not eat the food.

16. The answer is C. *(Schlesselman, pp 53–55.)* A statistically significant test ($p < 0.05$) rejects the null hypothesis, which states that no differences of effect will be found. A $p < 0.05$ indicates that a difference was found and there is <5 percent probability that it occurred by chance. No test of significance can determine causality or rule out errors or bias as the cause of an association. Neither can it imply clinical significance. A nonsignificant test may still have valuable clinical implications, such as the need for a larger, more involved study of a specific association.

17. The answer is E. *(Mausner, 2/e, pp 155–156.)* In *experimental* studies, the investigators determine exposure of the study and control groups to a suspected causal factor and measure responses in the two groups. In *observational* studies, investigators have no control over exposure to a suspected causal factor but can measure responses in those who are and are not exposed. In both types of studies, the attempt is made to use study and control groups similar in regard to all variables except exposure to the factor under study.

18. The answer is E. *(Schlesselman, pp 135–138.)* Misclassification bias—i.e., including people who do not really have the disease (controls) in the case groups—will tend to make the odds ratio falsely close to 1, rather than falsely high. (In the extreme example where misclassification is so bad that both case and control groups are really equal mixtures of cases and controls, the odds ratio necessarily would equal 1.) Recall bias could cause a falsely high odds ratio; it is potentially a problem when using maternal recall to investigate exposures associated with birth defects. It is less likely to be a problem for an exposure such as smoking than for an exposure that controls are more likely to forget. This study *is* a case-control study: the risk factor in this case is prenatal exposure to cigarette smoke. The placebo effect is of concern in unblinded intervention studies; it refers to the tendency of subjects to report improvement even when the treatment is not effective. It has no relevance to case-control studies.

19. The answer is B. *(Colton, pp 125–127.)* Since undescended testes are uncommon, the odds ratio in this study approximates the relative risk (risk ratio). The fact that the 95 percent confidence interval excludes 1.0 means that $p < 0.05$. Confidence intervals describe the range of values not significantly different from the observed value, with a type 1 error rate (alpha) of 1.0 minus the level of confidence. Thus, a 95 percent confidence interval shows the numbers that are not significantly different statistically from what was observed at the 5 percent level. The lower the level of confidence, the narrower the confidence interval, so a 90 percent confidence interval would be narrower than a 95 percent confidence interval, in this case excluding 1.0 for certain. Thus, if the study is accurate, it suggests that baby boys whose mothers smoke are 2.6 times as likely to have undescended testes.

20. The answer is D. *(Colton, pp 63–70.)* For two events or conditions, the probability that either will occur is the sum of their probabilities, minus the probability that both will occur. This is illustrated in the following figure:

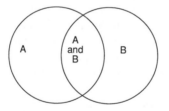

If we simply add the probability of A to the probability of B, the area labeled "A and B" will get counted twice. Therefore, the probability of (A and B) must be subtracted from the sum of the probabilities: p(A or B) = p(A) + p(B) − p(A and B). In this question, it is specifically stated that the two conditions are independent. When that is the case, the probability that both will occur is the product of their probabilities: p(A and B) = p(A) × p(B). The answer to this problem is 0.1 + 0.5 − (0.1)(0.5) = 0.55. Note that another common situation is when two conditions are mutually exclusive rather than independent (i.e., the probability that both will occur is zero). In this case, the probability that either one will occur is simply the sum of their probabilities. For example, if condition A were blue eyes and condition B brown eyes, the probability of either blue or brown eyes would be 0.60.

21. The answer is E. *(Schlesselman, pp 7–20.)* Case-control studies are well suited to studying rare disorders with multiple potential causes.

They are also quickly mounted and conducted and are less expensive than prospective studies. The large data base will enhance selection of a control group. The recent development of this data base eliminates it as a good source for long-term exposure data needed for a historical cohort study.

22. The answer is E. *(Schlesselman, p 69.)* Case-control studies do not involve an observational period, as do cohort studies. The disease in question has already occurred and the study is interested in examining antecedent exposures. Conducting field operations or pilot studies is also useful in planning and refining study protocols.

23. The answer is D. *(Ingelfinger, 2/e, pp 91–95.)* The normal (Gaussian) distribution is a symmetrical, bell-shaped distribution with many useful mathematical properties. Because it is symmetrical and unimodal, the mean is equal to the median and mode. It is entirely described by just two parameters: the mean and the standard deviation. The mean determines the location of the curve, the standard deviation how flat it is. As values get farther and farther from the mean, they become increasingly unlikely. Thus there are many more observations between 0 and 1 standard deviation from the mean than there are between 1 and 2 standard deviations from the mean. Approximately 68 percent of observations fall within 1 standard deviation of the mean, 95 percent within 2 standard deviations, and 99.7 percent within 3 standard deviations.

24. The answer is B. *(Ingelfinger, 2/e, p 723.)* Sensitivity and specificity are measures of how often a diagnostic test gives the correct answer. Sensitivity reflects the test's performance in people who *have* the disease, and specificity measures the test's performance in people who *do not have* the disease. These definitions can be illustrated as follows:

	Disease Present	Disease Absent
Test Positive	True Positive (TP)	False Positive (FP)
Test Negative	False Negative (FN)	True Negative (TN)

Sensitivity = TP / (TP + FN)   Specificity = TN / (TN + FP)

Among people who have the disease, there are two possibilities: either the test correctly identifies them (TP), or it falsely classifies them as negative (FN). Thus among those with disease, sensitivity measures how often the test gives the right answer. (A good way to remember sensitivity is by the initials PID: positive in disease.) Similarly, among people who do not have the disease, there are also two possibilities: either the test will correctly identify them as not having disease (TN), or it will falsely classify them as diseased (FP). Thus specificity measures how often the test gives the right answer among those who do not have the disease. (A good way to remember specificity is by the initials NIH: negative in health.)

As opposed to sensitivity and specificity, which measure the test's performance in groups of patients who do and do not have the disease, *predictive value* measures how often the test is right in patients grouped another way: by whether the test result is positive or negative. Thus, predictive value of a positive test is the proportion of positive tests that are true positives [TP / (TP + FP)], and predictive value of a negative result is the proportion of negative test results that are true negatives [TN / (TN + FN)].

But predictive value is a little tricky because it also depends on the *prevalence* of the disease in the population tested. In this case, Dr. Stewells assembled groups of 100 patients with and without cholera, and the prevalence is not given. Therefore, predictive value cannot be calculated in this question, and the correct answer is B, since specificity is 88 percent, not 12 percent.

25. The answer is C. *(Ingelfinger, 2/e, pp 7–23.)* In this study of 1000 patients with profuse diarrhea, 343 of them had cholera. Thus the prevalence of cholera (in this population) was 343/1000. (Note that this is not an incidence because we are measuring existing cases, rather than new cases that occur over a period of time.) The predictive value of a positive result can thus be directly determined as TP/(TP + FP) = 312/(312 + 79) = 80 percent. Similarly, the predictive value of a negative result is TN/(TN + FN) = 578/(578 + 31) = 95 percent. Note here that this predictive value refers to the predictive value of the test in patients *admitted to the hospital with profuse diarrhea.* Since prevalence data from the general population are still lacking, the usefulness of this test in the general population is undefined. Predictably, the positive predictive value of this test in an asymptomatic population will be less.

26. The answer is B. *(Ingelfinger, 2/e, pp 7–23.)* As the prevalence falls, more and more of those tested will *not* have cholera. This would change neither the sensitivity nor specificity of the test, which do not depend on disease prevalence, but would affect predictive value: as prevalence falls, predictive value of a positive result also falls, whereas predictive value of a negative result rises. This makes sense: As a disease becomes more and more unlikely, positive test results should be viewed with increasing skepticism, whereas negative results become increasingly believable.

27. The answer is A. *(Colton, p 257.)* Randomization is the use of a predetermined plan of allocation or assignment of subjects to treatment groups such that assignment occurs solely by chance. It is used to eliminate bias on the part of the investigator and the subject in the choice of treatment group. The goal of randomization is to allow chance to distribute unknown sources of biologic variability equally to the treatment and control groups. However, because chance does determine assignment, significant differences between the groups may arise, especially if the number of subjects is small. Therefore, whenever randomization is used, the comparability of the treatment groups should be assessed to determine whether or not balance was achieved.

28. The answer is B. *(Colton, pp 115–117.)* A p value of 0.60 indicates that the observed (or a greater) difference between the means could occur by chance as often as 6 times out of 10. This is not the same as saying that this result did occur by chance. Such a probability of chance is usually interpreted to mean that the result is not statistically significant. A value of p of 0.05 is the conventional upper limit of significance. However, even though p = 0.60, the null hypothesis of no difference between the means is not proved to be true. The most that can be said when the p value is not statistically significant is that the data are insufficient to cast doubt on the truth of the null hypothesis. If the samples were larger in size, the difference might be found to be statistically significant.

29. The answer is D. *(Mausner, 2/e, pp 156–159.)* The study described was a case-control study. In this type of study, people who have a disease (cases) are compared with people whom they closely resemble except for the presence of the disease under study (controls). Cases and controls are then studied for the frequency of exposure to a suspected risk factor. In case-control studies, the validity of inferences about the causal relationship between the exposure (cigarette smoking) and the disease (lung cancer) depends on how comparable the cases and controls are for all variables that may be related to both the risk factor and disease under study (e.g., age, sex, race, place of residence, and occupation).

30. The answer is B. *(Last, Maxcy-Rosenau, 13/e, p 16.)* Detecting fatal conditions that have no treatment or improved prognosis from early detection and intervention is not an effective use of time or money. Limited public resources are best spent on health conditions that have the most impact on public health. Studies that track and describe Alzheimer's disease, however, are valid epidemiologic research.

31–33. The answers are 31-D, 32-B, 33-E. *(Rothman, pp 311–313.)* The *excess risk* is the incidence in those exposed to the risk factors minus the incidence in those unexposed. Those, the excess risk from drinking among nonsmokers is $30 - 10 = 20$ cases per 10,000 person-years. Similarly, for smoking (among nondrinkers) it is $50 - 10 = 40$ cases per 10,000 person-years. The *relative risk* for smoking among nondrinkers is $50/10 = 5.0$, but the overall relative risk also depends on the relative risk in drinkers, which may be higher, lower, or the same. The overall relative risk also depends on the proportion of the population that drinks: the lower that proportion, the closer the overall relative risk will be to that of nondrinkers. To determine which risk factor is the cause of a greater number of cases (*population attributable fraction,* sometimes called *attributable risk*) requires knowledge of the prevalence of the risk factor, as well as its relative risk.

When there is more than one risk factor for a disease, it is important to compare the risk in those with both risk factors with that expected under different models of causation. Under an additive model, when risk factors are independent, *excess risks add.* Thus the excess risk for smoking and drinking would be $20 + 40 = 60$. To give an excess risk of 60 requires that $X = 70$.

Under a multiplicative model, when risk factors are independent, *relative risks multiply.* Thus the relative risk for patients with both risk factors should be $3 \times 5 = 15$. Thus X must be $15 \times 10 = 150$.

These questions demonstrate that determining the presence of independence, synergy, or antagonism among risk factors requires clear specification of whether one is dealing with an additive or multiplicative model of causation.

34. The answer is D. *(Mausner, 2/e, pp 43–45.)* Neither incidence nor prevalence rates of leukemia can be determined from the data given in the table without knowledge of the population at risk for leukemia and served by the study hospital. The data given provide numerators, but the lack of age-specific data on population prevents calculation of rates. The only conclusion (among those given in the question) that can be based on the data is that in the period 1970 to 1984 the number of children admitted to the hospital with a diagnosis of leukemia increased for the children 9 years old and under.

35. The answer is C. *(Hulley, pp 212–213.)* The idea of a randomized study is to compare groups of patients who get one drug with groups of patients who get another (or placebo). Such a comparison is called a *between-groups* comparison because one whole group is compared with another. The analysis described in this question illustrates a *within-group* analysis. Within-group analyses in randomized studies are often interesting but cannot provide convincing evidence of causality. Only comparisons between entire randomized groups take advantage of the randomization to provide strong evidence for causality. In fact, the difference in mortality between those who did and did not adhere to placebo was even greater: 15 percent versus 28 percent. Thus, something related to taking study medication (active or not) appears to have been a strong predictor of mortality.

36. The answer is D. *(Last, Maxcy-Rosenau, 13/e, p 30.)* The attributable risk percentage is a measure of the percentage of all deaths that can be directly attributed to the exposure being studied. The risk difference is the risk for those exposed minus the risk for those not exposed. The risk difference for smoking and lung cancer is 125 − 5, or 120, per 100,000. The attributable risk percentage is determined by dividing the risk difference by the risk for those who smoke, then multiplying by 100. The percentage of lung cancer deaths directly related to smoking is $(120/125) \times 100 = 96$ percent.

37. The answer is B. *(Ingelfinger, 2/e, pp 258–263.)* As a general rule, it is much easier to get a falsely negative result on a randomized blinded trial than a falsely positive result. The reason is that errors will tend to affect both treatment groups, making it harder to show a difference between them. Thus, in this question, inclusion of subjects without the ear effusion (who could not benefit from the intervention) and incorrect determination of which effusions resolved would both lead to falsely negative, not falsely positive results. Similarly, a small sample size is a reason for a falsely negative, but not a falsely positive result. Only chance (random error) or a breakdown in the blinding or randomization process would be causes of a falsely positive result.

38. The answer is A. *(Last, Maxcy-Rosenau, 13/e, p 32.)* A confidence interval is a range of possible values for the attribute that is being assessed and is designed in such a way that this range has a certain probability of including the true value. A 95 percent confidence interval, equivalent to $\alpha = 0.05$, will include the true value 95 percent of the time. The confidence interval reflects not only the relevant range of possibilities, but reflects sample size and statistical significance as well. A larger range indicates a smaller sample size. A confidence interval for a relative risk that includes 1.0 would indicate a nonsignificant statistical association (there is a 95 percent chance that the relative risks would be the same or 1.0). The p value only indicates the probability that the association occurs by chance. Statistical power only gives the probability of avoiding missing a true difference between exposure groups (type II, or B, error).

39. The answer is C. *(Mausner, 2/e, pp 200, 348–352.)* Sample size for a clinical trial depends on the frequency with which the outcome occurs in the control group, the magnitude of the effect that is to be detected, and the type 1 and type 2 error rates, alpha and beta. (A type 1 error occurs when the study erroneously finds a difference between two groups; a type 2 error is when the two groups really are different, but the study does not reach that conclusion.) An additional consideration in prospective studies, particularly those of long duration, is loss of follow-up, including mortality from causes not under investigation. The number of subjects required for the study is not affected by the prevalence of smoking because only smokers will be enrolled.

40. The answer is E. *(Last, Maxcy-Rosenau, 13/e, pp 22–24.)* Proposing measures of control and prevention should only take place after the investigation has defined the cause and determined the distribution of the population at risk. Although the exact sequence may vary, the ultimate purpose of an epidemiological investigation is to control a health problem in a community.

41. The answer is B. *(Last, Maxcy-Rosenau, 13/e, pp 24–26.)* A case-control study involves identifying two groups based on presence (case) or absence (control) of a disease. They are then compared as to their exposure histories. Many different exposures can be evaluated. A cohort study identifies two groups based on exposure to one hypothesized cause, those with exposure and those without. The subsequent rates of disease development are then compared. Only cohort studies can determine or compare rates. However, cohort studies are more lengthy, require larger numbers, and are more expensive than case-control studies.

42. The answer is D. *(Rothman, pp 64–68.)* The distribution of ABO blood type would be the same for matched controls of either sex; thus male controls are as valid as female controls. Use of males as controls would eliminate detection bias in the study. Detection bias would allow women with undiagnosed cervical cancer to serve as controls and thus confound any associations found between ABO blood type and cervical cancer. Inclusion of males as controls would not affect estimation of risk.

43. The answer is E. (*Last, Maxcy-Rosenau, 13/e, pp 42–44.*) Comparison of crude death rates of countries with different population compositions is fruitless. Adjusting both crude death rates to a standard population gives age-adjusted rates, which *can* be compared. Developed nations have higher crude death rates because a larger proportion of its population is elderly and thus has a higher probability of dying. Since rates account for population size, a larger population can be compared with a smaller one. Death rates are just one factor in evaluating health care systems.

44. The answer is E. (*Mausner, 2/e, pp 155, 312–316.*) In cohort studies, a group of subjects is defined on the basis of certain baseline characteristics and followed over time for the development of the disease (or other outcome) under study. The incidence of disease in subjects with various characteristics can then be compared with the incidence in subjects without those characteristics. If a suitable cohort can be identified from past records, a *retrospective* cohort study is possible. Cohort studies are not necessary to estimate prevalence. The prevalence of disease is the proportion of the population who have it at one point in time. Prevalence can be estimated from cross-sectional studies.

45. The answer is B. (*Hulley, pp 75–76.*) Because the association between the risk factor (use of smokeless tobacco) and the disease (oral lesions) is measured at a single point in time in a whole group of subjects, this is a *cross-sectional* study. A *case-control* study might be performed over a similar time period, but the sampling would be different: one sample would be selected from among those baseball players found to have oral lesions (the cases) and a separate sample would be selected from among those players whose mouths were normal (the controls). In a *cohort* study, the habits of a group of players initially free of the disease would be measured, and these players would be followed over time to see how many develop the lesions. A *clinical trial* involves allocation of the subjects by the investigator (usually randomly) to one of two or more treatment groups.

46. The answer is B. (*Last, Maxcy-Rosenau, 13/e, pp 27–28.*) This is a cross-sectional study. Cross-sectional studies allow one to estimate the *prevalence* (the number of existing cases at one point in time divided by the population at risk) but not *incidence* (number of new cases occurring over a period of time divided by the population at risk and the period of time at risk). The *prevalence* of mouth lesions is 80/110 (73 percent) in the users of smokeless tobacco.

47. The answer is B. *(Last, Maxcy-Rosenau, 13/e, pp 28–32.)* The odds ratio in this question is correct and likely to be highly statistically significant. Because the data are for two dichotomous variables and the expected value in each cell of the table is at least 5, the chi-square test could be used to determine the statistical significance of the data. However, when the disease is common (as is the case in this study), the odds ratio is very different from the risk ratio. Thus, while the odds ratio is 45.3, the risk ratio (actually, the prevalence ratio) is (80/110)/(2/36) = 13.1. Thus, users of smokeless tobacco are 13.1 (not 45.3) times as likely as nonusers to have mouth lesions. Misinterpretation of the odds ratio as a risk ratio when the disease is common is one of the most frequent statistical errors in the medical literature.

48. The answer is D. *(Last, Maxcy-Rosenau, 13/e, pp 28–32.)* Among those who have the risk factor, the proportion of those with the disease that can be explained by the risk factor is called the *attributable fraction* in the exposed. This statistic can be used clinically (as in this case), and the formula is easily memorized: $(RR - 1)/RR$. Recall that the relative risk of mouth lesions in users of smokeless tobacco attributable to smokeless tobacco is 12.1/13.1, or about 92 percent.

49. The answer is D. *(Ingelfinger, 2/e, pp 8–9.)* The choice of an optimal cutoff for a screening test often involves weighing the relative benefits of sensitivity and specificity. There is no set rule about which is the more important; rather, the decision must depend upon the consequences of false positive or false negative results. For example, because there is no good treatment for amyotrophic lateral sclerosis, a delay in diagnosis (or a missed diagnosis) caused by an insensitive test would be of little consequence. But since the diagnosis of ALS could end the search for a treatable cause of the patient's symptoms, a false positive result could be devastating. Thus for ALS, specificity is far more important than sensitivity. The situation is reversed for neonatal hypothyroidism, in which consequences of a false negative test (i.e., a child with hypothyroidism is missed by the test) are much worse than consequences of a false positive test (additional tests or even unnecessary thyroid hormone).

50. The answer is B. *(Benenson, 15/e, pp 499, 509.)* An *epidemic* is the occurrence of an illness, in a specific geographic area, that clearly exceeds the normal, expected incidence. *Hyperendemic* indicates a situation in which there is a persistent transmission of a disease among most of a population (as with malaria in certain parts of Africa). *Endemic* indicates the constant presence of a disease in a specific geographic area. *Enzootic* refers to the constant presence of a disease in animals in a specific geographic area. *Pandemic* refers to the worldwide spread of an epidemic disease.

51. The answer is B. *(Benenson, 15/e, pp 497, 501.)* The incubation period is the duration of time between exposure to an infectious agent and the appearance of the first manifestation of the disease. In contrast, the decubation period is the time from the disappearance of symptoms until recovery and the absence of infectious organisms. The communicable period designates the time when the infected person can transmit the infectious agent to another person.

52. The answer is C. *(Wilson, 12/e, pp 954–956.)* The importance of blinding, while it usually cannot be overemphasized, is not relevant in a study with total mortality as the end point: it is not possible to misclassify someone as alive when that person is really dead (except with fraudulent results). Power is not relevant in a study that shows a significant effect. In a randomized study, the percentages of patients who actually had myocardial infarctions should be similar in the two groups. Total mortality is a much more important end point than mortality from coronary heart disease, but long-term follow-up is absolutely essential in determining whether a therapy is useful. Perhaps the new agent simply postpones mortality by a few days or weeks.

53. The answer is A. *(Wilson, 12/e, p 1289.)* When considering whether to screen for a disease, the prevalence rather than the incidence of asymptomatic cases is relevant, since you will be interested in knowing what proportion of your patients have the disease at the time that you institute the screening policy. (The incidence would be relevant in determining how frequently to repeat the screening test.) The exact value of the specificity in particular is extremely important; a specificity of 98 percent would have a false positive rate of 2 percent, which is 20 times higher than if the specificity is 99.9 percent. No matter how inexpensive the test is, unless the survival rate of screened patients is substantially better than the survival rate for unscreened patients, the test will not be worthwhile (this could only be established with a randomized controlled trial).

54. The answer is B. *(Benenson, 15/e, p 501.)* The secondary attack rate of a disease is the ratio of the number of cases of a specified disease among persons exposed to index cases divided by the total number so exposed. According to the data, 400 cases of pertussis occurred among 4000 fully immunized children who were exposed to a sibling who had the disease. The secondary attack rate, as a percentage, among fully immunized children after household exposure is, therefore,

$$\frac{400}{4000} \times 100\% = 10\%$$

55. The answer is C. *(Greaves, Pediatr Infect Dis 2:284–286, 1983.)* The efficacy of vaccine, or the percentage reduction in the incidence of disease in vaccinated compared with unvaccinated subjects, is given by the expression

$$\text{Protection} = \frac{\text{incidence in unvaccinated} - \text{incidence in vaccinated}}{\text{incidence in unvaccinated}} \times 100$$

$$= \frac{(400/1000 - (400/4000)}{400/1000} \times 100\% = 75\%$$

56. The answer is E. *(Last, Maxcy-Rosenau, 13/e, pp 28–32.)* The relative risk is the ratio of the incidence rates of two groups who differ by some factor—in this instance, immunization status:

$$\frac{\text{Incidence rate among unimmunized children}}{\text{Incidence rate among fully immunized children}}$$

or

$$\frac{400 \text{ cases}/1000 \text{ exposed children}}{400 \text{ cases}/4000 \text{ exposed children}} = \frac{0.4}{0.1} = 4$$

57. The answer is D. *(Benenson, 15/e, p 501.)* The incidence of illness (as a percentage) is the total number of persons who have symptomatic illness divided by the total population at risk, and the calculation is (312 ÷ 614) × 100% = 50.8%.

58. The answer is C. *(Benenson, 15/e, p 501.)* The percentage of cases of German measles that were asymptomatic, or subclinical, is calculated by dividing the number of asymptomatic persons by the total number of infected persons. The calculation is $[207 \div (207 + 312)] \times 100\% = 39.9\%$.

59. The answer is E. *(Benenson, 15/e, p 501.)* Age-specific infection rates were 90 percent in all age groups 0 to 59 years of age, while the rate was 10 percent in persons over 60 years of age. The low attack rate in persons over 60 suggests that this age group had developed immunity to German measles as a result of prior exposure at least 60 years before—since there was uniform susceptibility in persons under 60.

60. The answer is E. *(Wilson, 12/e, p 1090.)* The exact proportion of deaths due to pulmonary embolism is not known and could only be determined by a study of a random sample of all persons who died. This would avoid the problem of selection bias (only certain persons undergo autopsies). The study should be large enough to avoid random error (perhaps the cited study found emboli in three of five autopsies), and the investigators should have careful and precise definitions of pulmonary embolism to avoid overdiagnosis of the condition. The association between pulmonary embolism and death may be due to confounding if some other factor causes both. Thus, pulmonary embolism, though present, may not be the cause of death. Lead-time bias refers to an apparent increase in survival among persons whose disease is detected by screening. For example, 5-year survival of cancer patients identified on screening might appear to be prolonged simply as a result of starting to count the survival time earlier in the course of disease.

61. The answer is A. *(Wilson, 12/e, p 947.)* (Notice that in this example, epidemiologic "jargon" is easier to understand than English!) A sensitive test is one that is positive in most patients with a disease. If the absence of a characteristic rules out a disease, then the test is sensitive; hardly anyone with the disease has a negative test. It is not possible to determine the specificity of this test, however, without knowing the proportion of patients *without* severe aortic stenosis who have calcification.

62. The answer is B. *(Rothman, p 79.)* The null hypothesis is the premise being tested by the study. It usually predicts that no difference between the two groups will be found (no effect). It is not used to calculate sample size. The final parameter needed to calculate sample size in addition to those listed is the exposure prevalence in the absence of disease.

63. The answer is C. *(Wilson, 12/e, pp 953, 992.)* Do not let the magic words "Bayesian reasoning" fool you—even a young man with this clinical history is likely to be having a myocardial infarction (MI). The vast majority of MIs, even in 35-year-old men, are due to atherosclerosis. While an elevated cholesterol would increase someone's risk of an MI, most patients with an MI will not have such a high cholesterol level; many will even have normal cholesterol levels. All the usual diagnostic tests, including measurement of creatine kinase MB isozymes, would be useful.

64. The answer is D. *(Wilson, 12/e, pp 5–11.)* In decision analysis, utilities refer to the relative values placed on various outcomes. For example, perfect health might be assigned a utility of 100, and death assigned one of 0. What, then, would the utility be for life with moderate back pain? With careful questioning, one finds that most patients place a higher value on life with disability than would be anticipated.

65. The answer is A. *(Last, Maxcy-Rosenau, 13/e, pp 34–35.)* Meta-analyses combine results from several studies and, through statistical methods, calculate an overall estimate of effect. Ecological studies use data based on groups of people rather than individuals. Associations observed on an aggregate level may not represent associations on an individual level (ecological bias or ecological fallacy).

66. The answer is C. *(Schlesselman, pp 20–25.)* Determination of the presence of a cause and its effect at the same time, such as on a cross-sectional survey, does not support causality. The cause must be shown to precede the effect in time. In some cases, the cause may be years in the past, such as with radiation exposure and thyroid cancer. In this case, these events would not be apparent at the same time, yet the relationship would be causal.

67–70. The answers are 67-B, 68-A, 69-D, 70-C. *(Colton, pp 40–41, 131–133, 137–139, 174–177.)* Use of the student t test to assess the difference between the mean systolic pressures of pregnant and nonpregnant women would be appropriate since the two groups are independent samples and the outcome variable is quantitative and approximately normally distributed.

In the study comparing the occurrence of hepatitis B surface antigen in medical and dental students, use of chi-square analysis would be appropriate because both the predictor and outcome variables are dichotomous; that is, students are classified by the presence or absence of the antigen and by medical or dental student status.

To compare the levels of blood glucose in rats to whom a drug was administered, analysis of variance would be appropriate because six different groups are to be analyzed (two sexes and three drugs). Analysis of variance will permit evaluation of the effects and interaction of sex and drug on the glucose level.

The paired t test is appropriate for comparing paired (e.g., before and after) measurements. Use of the regular (student two-sample) t test in this instance is inappropriate because the two samples are not independent—the same subjects are in each.

71–74. The answers are 71-B, 72-A, 73-E, 74-A. *(Hulley, pp 100–103. Sackett, p 147.)* Effect modification (also called "interaction") occurs when one factor modifies the effect of another on outcome. As an example, a high bilirubin seems to be a much stronger risk factor for bilirubin-induced brain damage if the baby is sick in other ways.

Confounding occurs when the association between two variables is distorted by the fact that both are associated with a third. For example, the association between coffee and lung cancer is distorted by smoking: among nonsmokers and smokers considered separately, coffee and lung cancer may be completely unrelated, but when the two groups are combined, an association appears to be present. Similarly, lead levels need to be related to IQ separately at each level of socioeconomic status to assure that the association is not due to confounding. The possibility that hyperactive children have high lead levels because they are hyperactive, rather than vice versa, is not confounding; it is simply a case in which the direction of causality is turned around (effect-cause).

Lead-time bias refers to a distortion of the apparent efficacy of a screening program.

75–78. The answers are 75-A, 76-C, 77-B, 78-E. *(Mausner, 2/e, pp 47, 49, 55–56, 149–152, 312, 317.)* The *point prevalence* is the proportion of people in a population who have a disease at a given point in time. The numerator is the number of existing cases of a disease; the denominator is the total population at risk of the disease at that point in time.

In order to compare rates of disease or death in two or more groups that differ substantially in age, sex, or racial composition, adjustment or standardization of the rates is necessary to remove the effects of those differences. The *standardized mortality or morbidity ratio* (SMR) is the ratio of the observed number to the expected number of deaths or cases of the disease. For example, age-specific rates of angina pectoris in nonsmokers can be applied to the age distribution of smokers to obtain the expected number of cases of angina pectoris in the smokers. The SMR of smokers for angina pectoris is the observed number of cases divided by the expected number so calculated.

The *incidence rate* is the number of new cases of a disease that occur in a period of time divided by the population at risk during that time.

The *relative risk* is the incidence of disease in subjects with a risk factor divided by the incidence in those in whom the factor is absent. (The denominator is *not* the incidence in the general population because then subjects *with* the risk factor would be included. If the risk factor is uncommon and the relative risk is close to 1.0, the error involved in using the general population for the denominator is small. However, other risk factors, e.g., a relative with CHD, are quite prevalent.) The term *relative risk* can be confusing when the risk factor has to do with being a *relative* of a patient; in this instance *risk ratio* is a preferable synonym.

79–83. The answers are 79-C, 80-E, 81-D, 82-B, 83-A. *(Wilson, 12/e, p 7.)* Although these terms are usually applied to epidemiologic studies, they are also applicable to examples from everyday life. Lead-time bias commonly refers to the apparent increase in life expectancy seen in patients who have their disease diagnosed with a screening test. The problem is that the screening test does not actually result in the patients' living any longer than they would have otherwise; the fact is simply that these patients are detected with the disease earlier in the disease's course. The same would be true of a study that found that anatomy students lived at the same address for a longer period of time than fourth-year medical students, most of whom move to start internships. The study would not be wrong, but any conclusions that suggested that anatomy students are more stable than fourth-year clerks would be meaningless.

Surveillance bias refers to overdetection of the disease of interest because one of the groups goes to the doctor (or has a diagnostic test) more often than does another group. For example, women who take postmenopausal estrogens presumably go to the doctor (and probably have mammograms) more frequently than women who do not; thus, women who take estrogens may be more likely to have breast cancers detected because of the increased surveillance. Similarly, you are more likely to find something that is lost in June (when you may be moving) than in March, when you are presumably in the middle of the term.

Recall bias classically refers to a situation in which persons with a disease are more likely to remember an exposure (say, to a toxic chemical) than persons who are healthy. This is part of a human tendency to look for explanations for bad outcomes—like failing an examination.

A type 1 error occurs when a result is found to be statistically significant by chance in a sample even though there is no effect in the population. In the case of answering the question correctly, the chance of a type 1 error is 20 percent because even if you did not know anything about this question, you would have a 1 in 5 chance of getting it correct. This could also be an example of misclassification bias. Misclassification bias usually occurs when someone without a disease is mistakenly classified as having the disease (for example, someone who dies suddenly of a pulmonary embolism may be misclassified as having died of a myocardial infarction). It can also refer to misclassification of the exposure status of a person; for example, a nonsmoker might be classified as a smoker because he or she checked the wrong box on a form. Medical school faculty commonly misclassify students; your best hope is to try to ensure that the misclassification is in your favor.

Power is the chance of finding an effect in your sample if it truly exists in the population. One problem with finding out that your friends have been out at the movies is that they may not tell you the truth (recall bias), or you may ask the wrong ones, such as those sitting next to you in the library (surveillance bias). So you can give yourself credit if you made one of those choices as well, assuming you understood what you were doing!

84–87. The answers are 84-B, 85-E, 86-A, 87-C. *(Mausner, 2/e, pp 54–55, 264, 280–281.)* The *case fatality rate* is a measure of the severity of the disease. It is a ratio of the number of deaths caused by a disease to the total number of cases of that disease and is usually expressed as a percentage. The *crude mortality* equals the total number of deaths from all causes during a year divided by the average population at risk during that year. It is usually expressed as the number of deaths per 1000 people. The *secondary attack rate* is a measure of the contagiousness of an infectious disease. The numerator is the number of cases of disease in contacts of the index case; the denominator is the number of contacts exposed to the index case during a specified period. Rates of disease are called *morbidity rates*.

88–91. The answers are 96-B, 97-A, 98-E, 99-B. *(Hulley, pp 99–108. Mausner, 2/e, pp 329–332.)* Matching is a way of selecting subjects that are comparable with respect to specific variables. For example, in a case-control study, a control could be selected that is the same age and sex as the case. It is thus a *sampling* strategy to achieve comparability among groups.

Stratification is an analysis strategy with the same purpose. Thus, after the study has been completed, the subjects can be stratified, i.e., divided into separate, relatively homogeneous strata, and the comparison between groups can occur within each stratum. For example, survival could be compared separately in different age strata, as in question 88. This might be important if the subjects with high renin levels were also older than the subjects with low levels, since a difference in survival between the two groups might be due to age, rather than to differing renin levels.

Age adjustment takes stratification by age one step further. After mortality (or another parameter) is calculated for specific age strata, it is combined in a weighted average to yield a single number. The weights used are the sizes of the different age strata in a standard population. Age adjustment is used more often for comparing mortality in populations with differing age structures.

Multivariate statistical analysis, like stratification, is an analysis technique for achieving comparability among groups. It involves *modeling* the associations between variables in order to allow their different effects to be isolated from each other. (For example, in multiple regression, the relationships between variables are modeled as a straight line.)

Survival analysis is a technique by which persons followed for variable lengths of time are counted according to the length of time they were followed. For example, in the cohort study of renin levels mentioned above, instead of simply comparing the proportions surviving 5 years, the cumulative probability of survival could be plotted for the two groups, and the two curves compared.

92–95. The answers are 92-D, 93-A, 94-B, 95-D. *(Colton, pp 6–7, 243–244.)* For proper comparison of the frequency of a disease in two groups, the rate of disease, not the number of cases, must be compared. The number of cases may reflect the age structure of the population served by the hospital. Age-specific attack rates that incorporate the number of cases in each age group, divided by the number of persons in each group, should be calculated.

In order to determine that an association between two conditions such as diabetes and obesity exists, an investigator must show that obesity is significantly more common in persons who have diabetes than in persons who do not have diabetes. The controls are necessary in order to test the significance of the association and must resemble the cases *ev. l absent, stand up !*

as closely as possible in all ways except for the absence of the disease under study.

Whenever considerable numbers of a cohort are lost to follow-up, doubts about the validity of the conclusions arise. Because death may be a major reason for loss to follow-up, the most conservative approach is to assume that everyone lost to follow-up has died. Unless, in this example, the death rate in the anxiety neurosis cohort was *still* no greater than that in the general population (after adding another 50 deaths for the 20 percent of the 250 patients lost to follow-up), the conclusions are suspect.

The conclusion in question 95 is invalid because of the lack of denominators to calculate the rate of bacterial endocarditis in different age groups. In addition, the autopsy series merely gives an estimate of the proportion of deaths in different age groups, not the frequency of occurrence of endocarditis with age. The autopsy series may also be invalid as a source of data from which to draw conclusions because of factors that determined whether an autopsy was performed.

96–99. The answers are 88-A, 89-B, 90-B, 91-A. *(Ehrlich, Pediatrics 70:665, 1982. Siegel, pp 315–344.)* One of the most commonly made statistical errors is use of tests that assume that each of the observations is independent when data sets violate that assumption. Be very suspicious that this assumption might be violated any time the denominators are greater than the number of study subjects. For example, in question 96, even though group sizes were 24 and 9, denominators for the proportions compared were 231 and 55. If observations are independent, it means that each observation gives the same amount of information. For dichotomous (yes/no) variables, as in this example, it means that the probability of a "yes" is the same for each observation. Returning to the example of urine cultures, since the overall proportion of positive cultures was 34/55 in the diversion group, it means that the best estimate of the probability that each culture will be positive should be 34/55. But what if one particular patient had received 20 of those cultures, and 19 had been positive? The best estimate of the probability that another culture from that person would be positive is 19/20, not 34/55. Thus, if one wishes to estimate the probability of a positive culture in an individual, not all the observations in the sample give the same amount of information: previous cultures on the same person would be more informative than cultures on others.

The situation is similar (though a bit more subtle) in question 99. Here the denominators are (appropriately) children, but once again, not all observations are independent. The trouble here is that all the subjects are in four classrooms, and if one child in the classroom develops chickenpox, other children in that class are much more likely to do so. For example, if by chance the one new contact with chickenpox happened to be in one of the control group classes, many people in that class would be infected. As was the case with urine cultures, if one wanted to estimate the probability that a specific child would get chickenpox, not all observations would be equally informative; observations on other members of the same class would be much more relevant.

Another very commonly made error is use of statistics that assume that the data are normally distributed when that assumption is false. This is the error in questions 97 and 98. The normal distribution is bell-shaped, symmetrical, and continuous. Data with a limited number of categories (such as parity) violate the assumption of normality, particularly if the mode is not somewhere near the middle category. The other main way in which the normality assumption is violated is by very skewed distributions, i.e., asymmetrical distributions that have some very extreme values on one side. Length of hospital stay is a good example: A single patient with a very complicated hospital course may tremendously affect the mean length of stay and its standard deviation in whichever group that patient is in. (Note that to some extent, these two effects cancel each other out because they tend to affect the p value in opposite directions. The statistical way of saying this is that the t test is fairly *robust* to violations of the assumption of normality.) A helpful rule is this: There should be equal numbers of values at the mean plus and minus 2 standard deviations. In questions 97 and 98, values of < 1.0 or 1.5 standard deviations below the mean were not possible: a negative length of stay or a negative number of children would result. (In each case the mean is less than 2.0 standard deviations from a lower limit for the variable.) Whenever the assumption of normality is not reasonable, and the sample size is not large, the data should be analyzed using a nonparametric technique, such as a rank sum test. In the example regarding length of hospital stay, it is quite possible that use of a nonparametric technique would lead to a lower p value, if, for example, there were a few patients with very long lengths of stay, as might be expected in a study of premature infants. Note that the assumption of a normally distributed variable is most important when the sample size is small. With large sample sizes (N > 100), the t test can be used even with very skewed variables because the central limit theorem applies.

100–103. The answers are 100-A, 101-D, 102-E, 103-C. *(Hulley, pp 204–205.)* If the probability of an event is p, the *odds* of the event are $p/(1 - p)$. The *odds ratio* is the ratio of the odds of exposure to the risk factor given disease (a/c) to the odds of exposure to the risk factor given no disease (b/d). To illustrate that the odds of exposure given disease are a/c, the probability of exposure given disease is $p = a/(a + c)$. So $(1 - p) = c/(a + c)$, and the odds are $[a/(a + c)]/[c/(a + c)]$, and the $(a + c)$'s cancel out to give a/c. The odds ratio, therefore, is $(a/c)/(b/d)$, which equals ad/bc.

Odds ratios are mainly used in case-control studies, from which relative risk cannot be calculated directly. When the disease is rare, the odds ratio closely approximates the relative risk. However, the study in the example is a cohort study, so relative risk can be calculated directly from the table. It is equal to the risk (incidence) of suicide in those who served in Vietnam divided by the risk in those who served elsewhere, or $[a/(a + b)]/[c/(c + d)]$.

Excess risk is defined as the *difference* between the risk in those with the risk factor and those in whom it is absent. Whereas the relative risk and odds ratio are unitless (since any measurement of time in the denominators cancel out), the excess risk must have an explicit or implied time period on the denominator. In this example, $a/(a + b) - c/(c + d)$ represents the excess risk of suicide in Vietnam veterans over a 5-year period; it is five times as big as the excess risk for a 1-year period. Thus, if the yearly risk of suicide was 0.2 percent in Vietnam veterans and 0.1 percent in other veterans, the relative risk would be 2.0, and the excess risk (risk difference) 0.1 percent per year, or 0.5 percent over the 5-year period.

The overall incidence of suicide (per 5 years) in the study is simply the number of suicides $(a + c)$ divided by the population at risk $(a + b + c + d)$. (Note that a more precise way to measure the incidence, relative risk, and so on would be to use person-years at risk on the denominators, but this leads to greater computational and conceptual complexity.)

104–107. The answers are 104-C, 105-E, 106-A, 107-D. *(Hulley, pp 24– 25.)* *Simple random sampling* is a process in which individuals are sampled independently, and each individual of the population has an equal probability of being selected.

In *cluster sampling,* groups of people (e.g., families, school classes) are selected at random, and then everyone in those groups is sampled. A common analytic mistake is to pretend that subjects obtained in a cluster sample were obtained in a simple random sample. This can lead to incorrect results because the subjects are not sampled independently.

Systematic sampling is a process that first requires the arrangement of the group to be sampled in some kind of order. Then individuals are selected systematically throughout the series on the basis of a predetermined sampling fraction or constant determinant, for example, every fifth, tenth, or hundredth person in the ordered group. Although systematic sampling may seem almost the same as simple random sampling, it is much less desirable. For example, sampling every other subject from a list in which husbands' and wives' names appear next to each other (e.g., an alphabetical list) will bias the sample—if husbands were always first, the sample might include no wives and would rarely include both persons in a married couple.

In *stratified sampling,* a population is divided into subgroups based on defined characteristics such as age, sex, or severity of illness, or any combination of these; then random samples are selected from each subgroup.

In *paired sampling,* or *matching,* selection of one or more controls for each case is based on age, sex, time, time sequence, geographic location, or some other defined relationship to the case. For example, selection could be based on the next patient admitted after each case, the sibling nearest in age to each case, or the person who lives closest geographically to each case.

108–112. The answers are 108-D, 109-E, 110-B, 111-E, 112-E. *(Wilson, 12/e, p 7.)* The easiest (and best) way to answer problems like this is to write out the appropriate two-by-two table. Since we were not told how many women were tested, we can just make up a number—say, 200. We are told that half have a positive test:

	Infection	No Infection	
Test Positive	?	?	100
Test Negative	?	?	100
			200

The next task is to fill in the remaining boxes. We are told that 45 percent of those with a positive test are infected with chlamydia:

	Infection	No Infection	
Test Positive	45	55	100
Test Negative	?	?	100
			200

and that 95 percent of those with a negative test are free of the disease:

	Infection	No Infection	
Test Positive	45	55	100
Test Negative	5	95	100
			200

This now allows us to say that for 200 women in the community, the following two-by-two table would be correct:

	Infection	No Infection	
Test Positive	45	55	100
Test Negative	5	95	100
	50	150	200

We can now determine the test's operating characteristics (sensitivity and specificity) and the other parameters. Sensitivity is simply the proportion of women with chlamydia who will have a positive test (remember: *PID* = *P*ositive *i*n *D*isease), or 45/50 = 90 percent. Specificity is the proportion of women without chlamydia who will have a negative test (remember: *NIH* = *N*egative *i*n *H*ealth), or 95/150 = 63 percent. The prevalence of the disease is simply the proportion of women with chlamydia, or 50 out of 200 = 25 percent. The predictive value of a positive test is the proportion of women with a positive test who have chlamydia; we were already told that this was 45 percent. Likewise, the predictive value of a negative test is the proportion of women with a negative test who do not have chlamydia; we were already told that this was 95 percent.

113–116. The answers are 113-B, 114-D, 115-A, 116-E. *(Colton, pp 28–31.)* Mean, median, and mode are all measures of central tendency, while variance, standard deviation, and range are measures of dispersion. In figure B, both distributions appear normally shaped, and they center on the same point, but curve 2 has greater variance because it is more spread out. Figure D, in contrast, shows two distributions with the same variance, but different means. In figure A, both the centers and the shapes of the curves differ. Curve 1 is skewed to the right, which means it has more of a tail on the right side.

Remember that the value that occurs most commonly (i.e., the highest point on the curve) is the mode, so choice E represents "pi a la mode"—a very tasty dessert.

117–120. The answers are 117-C, 118-A, 119-B, 120-D. *(Browner, JAMA 257:2459–2463, 1987. Michael, pp 31–38, 91–95, 105–112.)* A type 2 error occurs when a study fails to reject the null hypothesis (of no effect) when it is in fact false. Any time a study fails to achieve statistical significance, a crucial question to ask is whether the study had enough subjects. Although 500 subjects per group followed for 5 years seems like a large number, only a tiny minority (perhaps 10 per group) would be expected to have a myocardial infarction. Thus the sample size in this instance may have been inadequate to detect a meaningful difference between the groups.

The ecologic fallacy occurs when associations among groups of subjects are mistakenly assumed to hold for individuals. Thus, although among communities high rates of condom use may be associated with higher fertility rates (perhaps because condom use acts as a marker for sexual activity in general), among those who use the condoms, the fertility rate could in fact be zero.

A type 1 error occurs when, just by chance, a statistically significant difference between groups is found. Studies attempting to correlate multiple risk factors with multiple diseases (particularly when there is no good biologic reason to suspect an association) are especially prone to type 1 errors. Looking for associations separately in different subgroups compounds the problem.

Selection bias occurs when the subjects selected for the study are somehow not representative of the population from which they come. One trouble with selecting spouses for controls is that one's spouse is much more likely to share one's smoking habits than a person from the general population. Thus, since patients with lung cancer will be mostly smokers, smokers will be overrepresented among the controls, and smoking will look like a weaker risk factor than it really is.

121–125. The answers are 121-A, 122-C, 123-E, 124-B, 125-D. *(Last, Dictionary, 2/e, p 80.)* The scale of measurement is an important determinant of the amount of information in a variable and the type of statistical analysis that can be used. Dichotomous variables (like sex) have only two possible values. Some variables may be artificially dichotomized, with subsequent loss of information. For example, a patient either survives 5 years or not; thus survival to 5 years is an example of a dichotomous variable. The variable could be made more informative, however, if the actual number of months of survival was specified.

Nominal variables have more than two possible values, but no intrinsic ordering. Race is the classic example; medical specialties also have no intrinsic ordering. Nominal and ordinal are often confused. Just remember *nominal* for *no ordering*.

Ordinal variables are intrinsically ordered, but not in a quantitative way that allows one to say that there is a natural numerical distance between possible values. Thus one value cannot really be subtracted from another. Examples are qualitative judgments like "worse, same, better" or "never, sometimes, always." Remember, ordinal means *ordered*.

Interval scales are ordered, but with real numerical units; they can be subtracted from each other. An example is dates of birth: they are intrinsically ordered and subtracting them gives meaningful numbers, but there is no intrinsic zero to the scale, so that dividing them does not make sense—one date of birth cannot be twice as big as another.

Ratio scales are measurements in relation to a clear zero point. Thus, measurements on ratio scales can be meaningfully divided by each other. For example, one baby may weigh twice as much as another or have twice as high a platelet count. Absolute temperature is measured on a ratio scale, whereas temperature in Fahrenheit or Celsius is measured on an interval scale.

126–130. The answers are 126-A, 127-A, 128-A, 129-E, 130-D. *(Sackett, pp 59–100.)* Answering the first three of these questions is easiest if the results of Dr. Blues' research are displayed in a two-by-two table:

	Depressed	Not Depressed
Positive Blues test	80	80
Negative Blues test	20	320
Total	100	400

The sensitivity of a test is defined as the proportion of persons with a disease who have a positive test (positive in disease = PID): in this case, 80 out of 100, or 80 percent. This is the same as the likelihood that a person with depression will have a positive Blues test. The specificity of a test is defined as the proportion of persons without a disease who have a negative test (negative in health = NIH): in this case, 320 out of 400, or 80 percent.

The likelihood that someone with a positive test has the disease—known as the positive predictive value (PV +) of a test—depends upon how prevalent the disease is. By definition,

PV + = true positives ÷ total positives
    = true positives ÷ (true positives + false positives)
    = (sensitivity × prevalence) ÷ [(sensitivity × prevalence) + (1 − specificity) × (1 − prevalence)]
    = (0.8 × 0.01) ÷ [(0.8 × 0.01) + (0.2 × 0.99)] = 3.9%

The Blues test would not be very useful in diagnosing depression if applied to the general population. It might be useful in ruling out depression if negative, however. The likelihood that someone with a negative test has the disease equals 100 percent minus the likelihood that someone with a negative test does *not* have the disease. This latter quantity is known as the negative predictive value (PV −) and is defined as

PV − = true negatives ÷ total negatives
    = true negatives ÷ (true negatives + false negatives)
    = [specificity × (1 − prevalence)] ÷ [specificity × (1 − prevalence) + (1 − sensitivity × prevalence)]
    = (0.8 × 0.99) ÷ [(0.8 × 0.99) + (0.2 × 0.01)] = 99.7%

Since the likelihood that someone with a negative test is *not* depressed is 99.7 percent, the likelihood that someone with a negative test is depressed is (1 − 99.7 percent) or 0.3 percent. (A shortcut: Since we know that the overall prevalence of depression is only 1 percent, someone with a *negative* Blues test must be even less likely to be depressed than that!)

Epidemiology of Health and Disease

DIRECTIONS: Each question below contains five suggested responses. Select the **one best** response to each question.

131. Which of the following statements about aortic dissection is true?

(A) Almost all patients with aortic dissection have elevated serum cholesterol levels (> 240 mg/dL)
(B) Aortic dissection is the major cause of mortality in patients with Marfan's syndrome
(C) There is an increased incidence of aortic dissection in patients with Gaucher's disease
(D) There is approximately a 10 percent operative mortality from emergency surgery for dissection of the ascending aorta
(E) Acute aortic dissection is usually asymptomatic

132. The incidence of nosocomial (hospital-associated) infections among patients admitted to general hospitals in the United States is

(A) less than 1 percent
(B) 1 to 4 percent
(C) 5 to 10 percent
(D) 11 to 15 percent
(E) greater than 15 percent

133. In country A there are 35 new cases of breast cancer per 100,000 adult women per year; in country B the number is 90 per 100,000. Which of the following is the most likely explanation?

(A) Women in country A have a much higher rate of nursing their infants
(B) Women in country A are less likely to smoke cigarettes
(C) Women in country A receive more frequent preventive care, such as mammography
(D) Treatment is much more successful in country A
(E) Women in country A are younger

134. Studies in the epidemiology of appendicitis have shown that

(A) it affects girls nearly three times as frequently as boys
(B) its incidence is highest in the sixth and seventh decades of life
(C) its incidence is decreasing in the Western world
(D) its mortality is increasing in the Western world
(E) it affects about 1 in 1000 pregnancies

135. Correct statements about infant mortality include all the following EXCEPT

(A) the numerator is the number of infants who die before their first birthday for a given year
(B) the denominator is the number of births in a year
(C) in the United States, the difference in infant mortality between whites and blacks is 100 percent
(D) the rate is expressed per 1000 births
(E) the most important cause of postneonatal mortality is the sudden infant death syndrome

136. True statements about complications of appendicitis include all the following EXCEPT

(A) there is at least a 70 percent incidence of appendiceal perforation among patients with appendicitis who are under 2 years of age
(B) there is a 30 percent incidence of appendiceal perforation among patients with appendicitis who are over 70 years of age
(C) the incidence of perforation is higher in patients with leukocytosis ($> 20,000$ cells per microliter)
(D) surgical mortality is about 0.1 percent in the absence of perforation
(E) surgical mortality is about twice as high in the presence of perforation

137. Chickenpox is associated with

(A) a high case fatality rate
(B) congenital malformations in 10 percent of offspring of infected mothers
(C) a high reinfection rate
(D) a long prodromal period
(E) Reye syndrome

138. Giardiasis occurs on a worldwide basis and is associated with all the following EXCEPT

(A) waterborne transmission
(B) asymptomatic carriage
(C) bloating, abdominal cramps, and diarrhea
(D) invasion of colonic mucosa
(E) transmission from person to person

139. The newborn with cytomegalovirus (CMV) infection at birth most commonly presents with

(A) hepatosplenomegaly
(B) hepatitis
(C) thrombocytopenia
(D) cerebral calcifications
(E) no symptoms

140. Factors that are more characteristic of childhood-onset asthma than adult-onset asthma include

(A) a 2:1 ratio of females to males
(B) an association with a history of eczema
(C) normal levels of IgE in the serum
(D) lack of response to provocation with inhaled antigens
(E) lack of seasonal variation in severity of symptoms

141. Which of the following bacteria is the most common cause of bacterial meningitis in children 3 months to 6 years of age in the United States?

(A) *Streptococcus pneumoniae*
(B) Group B *Streptococcus hemolyticus*
(C) *Haemophilus influenzae* type b
(D) *Escherichia coli* K1
(E) *Neisseria meningitidis*

142. The bacteria that are involved in nosocomial infections are transmitted most often by

(A) airborne matter
(B) fomites
(C) exposure to a common source
(D) indwelling catheters
(E) direct contact via hands

143. All the following are clearly associated with acute episodes of asthma EXCEPT

(A) emotional stress
(B) elevated ozone concentrations
(C) aspirin
(D) caffeinated beverages
(E) upper respiratory infections

144. All the following statements about unintentional injuries in the United States are true EXCEPT

(A) nonfatal, unintentional injuries that required medical treatment affected an estimated 1 in 4 persons in 1987

(B) males have a higher death rate due to injuries

(C) falls account for the majority of fatal injuries in older adults

(D) injuries are the second leading cause of death in children

(E) motor vehicle accidents account for more than half of the deaths from unintentional injuries

145. Which is the most common site of nosocomial infections?

(A) Surgical wound

(B) Respiratory tract

(C) Blood stream

(D) Urinary tract

(E) Gastrointestinal tract

146. Which of the following is a true statement about homicide in the United States?

(A) Homicide is the leading cause of death for males 15 to 24 years of age

(B) Homicide is the twelfth leading cause of death for Americans

(C) The majority of homicides are committed during the perpetration of another felony or crime

(D) The lifetime risk of death from homicide is 1 in 100 for white males

(E) None of the above

147. A major complication of transfusion of blood and blood products has been the development of posttransfusion hepatitis. Research indicates that

(A) most cases of posttransfusion hepatitis are due to infection with hepatitis B virus

(B) the risk of posttransfusion hepatitis is highest following transfusions of albumin or immune globulin

(C) about 5 to 10 percent of patients who received blood or blood products developed posttransfusion hepatitis

(D) no screening test is available to detect blood that may transmit hepatitis C virus

(E) almost all cases of posttransfusion hepatitis are asymptomatic

148. Correct statements about obesity include all the following EXCEPT

(A) a woman whose body fat is greater than 30 percent of her total body mass is obese

(B) the average body weights of American men and women are increasing with no proportionate change in stature

(C) sedentariness appears to be the most important cause of obesity in Western populations

(D) obesity is a major risk factor for coronary heart disease

(E) genetic factors contribute to obesity

149. True statements about the epidemiology of cancer in the U.S. include all the following EXCEPT

(A) about 1.5 million cases of cancer develop each year
(B) cancer is responsible for about 20 percent of U.S. deaths
(C) one in three Americans will develop cancer in his or her lifetime
(D) the 5-year survival with cancer is about 50 percent
(E) lung cancer is the most common form of cancer in the U.S.

150. The parameter that can be used to obtain the best estimate of the prevalence of dental caries is

(A) the calculus index
(B) the malocclusion index
(C) the decayed, missing, or filled rate
(D) the oral hygiene index
(E) none of the above

151. Correct statements concerning upper respiratory infections include which of the following?

(A) Summertime outbreaks of illness characterized by fever, pharyngitis, and conjunctivitis have most frequently been associated with paramyxovirus infection
(B) Treatment with penicillin hastens recovery in children with streptococcal pharyngitis
(C) Patients with viral upper respiratory infections are generally most infectious the day before their symptoms begin
(D) The most common identifiable cause of pharyngitis is adenovirus
(E) None of the above

152. Studies of coronary artery bypass grafting have shown that all the following are true EXCEPT

(A) operative mortality is higher in women than in men
(B) operative mortality is higher in persons with diabetes
(C) operative mortality is approximately 1 percent in persons with normal left ventricular function
(D) when adjusted for severity of disease, there is little variation in operative mortality for surgery performed by different board-certified surgeons
(E) surgery reduces or eliminates angina in about 85 percent of patients

153. Which statement about obesity is correct?

(A) Osteoarthritis is less common among obese persons because of decreased activity
(B) In a normal person, 300 calories of excess carbohydrate will lead to the same weight gain as 300 calories of excess fat
(C) Obese persons are significantly less active than non-obese persons
(D) The apparent association between obesity and hypertension is probably due to the use of inappropriately small blood pressure cuffs in the obese subjects
(E) None of the above

154. Correct statements concerning breast-feeding include which of the following?

(A) The incidence of infections is greater in breast-fed than in bottle-fed infants
(B) Breast milk is frequently insufficient in quantity
(C) Iron deficiency anemia is less frequent in infants fed cow's milk
(D) Significant quantities of immunoglobulins are provided by breast milk
(E) None of the above

155. All the following statements about the epidemiology of breast cancer in women are true EXCEPT

(A) in the U.S., the cumulative lifetime probability of dying from breast cancer is about 4 percent
(B) 70 to 80 percent of all breast cancers occur in patients without identifiable risk factors
(C) the risk of developing breast cancer is highest for women over 75 years of age
(D) first-degree relatives of patients with breast cancer have a tenfold increased risk of developing breast cancer
(E) the incidence of breast cancer is highest in affluent, Westernized countries

156. All the following statements about coronary heart disease in the U.S. are true EXCEPT

(A) coronary heart disease is the most common cause of death in women after age 45
(B) coronary heart disease is the leading cause of death in men after age 35
(C) angina is a more frequent presentation in women than in men
(D) the incidence of myocardial infarction due to coronary heart disease increases fivefold from 40 to 60 years of age in all persons
(E) about 5 million Americans have coronary heart disease

157. Which of the following statements about colon cancer is true?

(A) It is two times more common in smokers
(B) There is an increased incidence of the disease in alcoholics
(C) Genetic factors are not believed to contribute to the development of colon cancer
(D) It is the second leading cause of cancer death in males
(E) High intake of dietary fiber increases the incidence of colon cancer

158. Among patients with intermittent claudication, all the following statements are true EXCEPT

(A) about 50 percent eventually require amputation if they do not undergo vascular reconstruction
(B) the leading cause of death is coronary heart disease
(C) about 50 percent have significant coronary artery disease at the time of presentation
(D) prognosis is worse in patients with diabetes
(E) cigarette smoking is the most powerful risk factor

159. Which of the following epidemiologic statements about gastric cancer is true?

(A) The incidence of gastric cancer has been decreasing worldwide
(B) Annual mortality for gastric cancer has been increasing over the last 40 years in the U.S.
(C) The incidence of gastric cancer is higher in smokers
(D) The incidence in women is twice that in men
(E) The incidence is higher in persons with a history of benign gastric ulcer

160. Premature loss of life can be defined as years of life lost due to a disease before the age of 65 years. The leading cause of premature loss of life in the U.S. is

(A) coronary heart disease
(B) cancer
(C) stroke
(D) congenital heart disease
(E) none of the above

161. All the following statements about disabling visual disorders are true EXCEPT

(A) cataracts cause between one-third and one-half of the cases of blindness in the world
(B) glaucoma is the most important cause of blindness among blacks in the U.S.
(C) proliferative retinopathy is the most common cause of blindness among persons with type I (juvenile-onset, insulin-dependent) diabetes
(D) persons with severe myopia are at an increased risk of retinal detachment
(E) trachoma is the most common cause of retinal detachment worldwide

162. Compared with the general population, all the following patients are at an increased risk of cobalamin (B$_{12}$) deficiency EXCEPT

(A) a 40-year-old man with a history of ingestion of lye at age 20
(B) a 20-year-old woman with a history of Graves' disease
(C) a 60-year-old man with a brother with pernicious anemia
(D) a 70-year-old woman with nontropical sprue
(E) a 30-year-old Scandinavian man who eats raw fish

163. Which of the following statements about microcytic anemia in the U.S. is true?

(A) It usually has a genetic cause in black children
(B) It is rarely caused by a dietary deficiency in men
(C) It is rarely caused by a dietary deficiency in women
(D) It is common in children with pinworm infestation
(E) It is not associated with pica

164. All the following are independently associated with prognosis in colon cancer EXCEPT

(A) size of the tumor
(B) abnormal DNA content (aneuploidy) in tumor cells
(C) number of involved lymph nodes
(D) poorly differentiated histology
(E) tumor in pericolonic fat

165. The ratio of the prevalence of type I (insulin-dependent) diabetes mellitus to type II (non-insulin-dependent) diabetes mellitus in the U.S. is about

(A) 1:1
(B) 1:4
(C) 1:9
(D) 4:1
(E) 9:1

166. A characteristic demographic feature of rheumatoid arthritis is an incidence ratio of 1:3 that applies to

(A) male:female
(B) blacks:whites
(C) rural:urban inhabitants
(D) high:low socioeconomic status
(E) Western:Eastern cultures

167. Possible risk factors for the development of colon cancer include all the following EXCEPT

(A) diets high in animal fat
(B) irritable bowel syndrome
(C) inflammatory bowel disease
(D) familial polyposis
(E) ureterosigmoidostomy

168. Which of the following statements about valvular heart disease is true?

(A) Coronary artery disease is the most common cause of aortic stenosis in the U.S.
(B) The incidence of rheumatic heart disease in the U.S. has been decreasing for the past 10 years
(C) Most persons with a history of rheumatic fever are immune to recurrence during group A streptococcal epidemics
(D) Most patients with mitral valve prolapse remain asymptomatic for their entire lives
(E) None of the above

169. Cystic fibrosis is a genetic disorder of exocrine gland function. All the following statements about cystic fibrosis are true EXCEPT

(A) it is the most common lethal genetic disease in whites in the U.S.
(B) it is inherited as an autosomal recessive trait
(C) about 1 in 20 whites are heterozygous for the gene
(D) the diagnosis can be confirmed by demonstrating an absence of chloride in the sweat
(E) the median survival rate for patients with cystic fibrosis is about 20 years

170. Asthma is characterized by which of the following?

(A) Onset before age 40 in about 95 percent of cases
(B) Persistently abnormal forced expiratory volume in 1 s (FEV_1)
(C) Greater frequency in girls than boys
(D) Frequent family history of atopy
(E) None of the above

171. The epidemiology of cystic fibrosis indicates that

(A) about 1 in 200 white Americans carries the gene responsible for the disease

(B) there is an elevated gene frequency among the Amish

(C) antenatal diagnosis is not possible

(D) median survival after birth is about 8 years

(E) about 40 percent of men with cystic fibrosis are infertile

172. Which of the following statements about emphysema is true?

(A) There is a definitive clinical diagnosis of the disease

(B) The majority of persons with emphysema are symptomatic

(C) Flow rates on pulmonary function tests resemble those seen in chronic bronchitis

(D) It is equally prevalent in light and heavy smokers

(E) It is associated with the chronic inhalation of coal dust

173. Studies of estimated mortality related to birth control in premenopausal women in the United States have shown that

(A) at all ages, mortality is greater among women using no contraception than among women using oral contraceptives

(B) the mortality associated with the use of abortion is less than birth-related mortality at all ages

(C) death rates associated with the use of intrauterine devices (IUDs) are about ten times higher in older than in younger women

(D) smokers who use birth control pills are at about a 15 percent higher mortality risk

(E) the highest birth-related death rates are seen among teenagers

174. Studies of musculoskeletal disorders in the U.S. have found that all the following statements are true EXCEPT

(A) they are a more common cause of limitation of activity than is cardiovascular disease

(B) back or spine impairments are the most common type

(C) 60 to 80 percent of the population experiences back pain at some time during their lives

(D) persons who engage in heavy manual work have a greater risk of suffering low back pain than persons who work at sedentary jobs

(E) lower back x-rays and medical examinations are useful ways to screen for workers at high risk of sustaining on-the-job back injuries

175. Which of the following statements about bronchiectasis is true?

(A) It is uncommon in childhood

(B) It is manifested by cough

(C) It is rarely accompanied by fever

(D) It is usually a primary disorder

(E) It is usually a self-limited problem

176. Studies of the epidemiology of cutaneous drug reactions have shown which of the following?

(A) The incidence of cutaneous drug reactions is highest in the elderly

(B) Urticaria is the most common skin manifestation

(C) Cutaneous drug reactions usually occur about 2 to 3 weeks following initial exposure

(D) The most common drugs involved are antihypertensive medications

(E) None of the above

177. International studies of cardiovascular disease have shown which of the following?

(A) Death rates due to coronary artery disease vary by less than 25 percent from country to country

(B) The death rate due to coronary artery disease is higher in the U.S. than in any European country

(C) The death rate due to coronary artery disease is similar in the U.S. and Japan

(D) The death rate due to coronary artery disease in the U.S. is declining

(E) Coronary artery disease is the leading cause of adult death in industrialized countries

178. Which of the following 60-year-old patients is most likely to have a stroke within a year?

(A) A male smoker
(B) A man with hypertension
(C) A man with an asymptomatic carotid bruit
(D) A woman with a recent transient ischemic attack
(E) A woman with diabetes mellitus

179. Which of the following statements about elderly Americans is true?

(A) Most of the difference in life expectancy between men and women is due to unalterable genetic factors
(B) Although there are more elderly women than men, fewer elderly women live alone
(C) A woman is less likely to be institutionalized in a nursing home than is a man
(D) Only 5 percent of elderly Americans are institutionalized at any one time
(E) The number of persons older than 65 years of age is expected to increase by nearly 15 percent in the next 40 years

180. The incidence of cholelithiasis (gallstones) is increased in all the following EXCEPT

(A) persons with diabetes
(B) persons with chronic hemolytic anemia
(C) persons with hypercholesterolemia
(D) persons who are obese
(E) women

181. Which of the following statements about systemic lupus erythematosus (SLE) is true?

(A) It is more common in whites than blacks
(B) The incidence increases with age
(C) It is approximately ten times more common in women than men
(D) The diagnosis requires a positive antinuclear antibody (ANA) test
(E) It is the most common cause of arthritis in women less than 35 years of age

182. Compared with the general population, all the following patients are at an increased risk of folate deficiency EXCEPT

(A) a 20-year-old man with sickle cell anemia
(B) a 20-year-old woman who is a strict vegetarian
(C) a 60-year-old man on hemodialysis
(D) a 70-year-old woman who drinks a quart of gin a day
(E) a 30-year-old man with tropical sprue

183. Compared with persons without kidney disease, patients on chronic dialysis for renal failure have an increased incidence of all the following EXCEPT

(A) infection with *Mycobacterium tuberculosis*
(B) infection with hepatitis B
(C) suicide
(D) coronary heart disease
(E) hypernephroma

184. The risk of developing cataracts is increased among all the following persons EXCEPT those with

(A) type I (insulin-dependent) diabetes
(B) a history of congenital rubella
(C) type II (non-insulin-dependent) diabetes
(D) an occupational exposure to video display terminals
(E) an occupational exposure to ultraviolet radiation

185. Which of the following is a risk factor for the development of hemophilia?

(A) HLA-B15
(B) Iron deficiency
(C) Hepatitis B surface antigen (HBsAg)
(D) Benzene exposure
(E) None of the above

186. There has been increasing age-adjusted mortality in the past 25 years from cancer of the

(A) lung
(B) uterus
(C) prostate
(D) testis
(E) stomach

187. Primary hepatocellular carcinoma (hepatoma) is

(A) more common in persons with chronic liver disease
(B) more common in women
(C) more common in persons with gallstones
(D) associated with cigarette smoking
(E) responsible for 10 percent of all cancers in Africa and Asia

188. Seroepidemiologic studies of infection with herpes simplex virus (HSV) have shown that

(A) infection with HSV-2 is more common than infection with HSV-1
(B) infection with one type of HSV provides protection against infection with the other type
(C) HSV-2 is only infectious during the symptomatic phase
(D) it is possible to differentiate HSV-1 from HSV-2 antibodies
(E) genital HSV-2 infection is less likely to reactivate than genital HSV-1 infection

189. A familial aggregation pattern exists for cancer of all the following organs EXCEPT

(A) breast
(B) retina
(C) colon
(D) larynx
(E) skin

190. All the following statements about the relationship between marital status and cancer are true EXCEPT

(A) the risk of cancer of the cervix is higher in married women compared with single women
(B) the risk of cancer of the cervix is lower in women who marry late in life than in women who marry earlier
(C) the risk of breast cancer is higher in single than in married women
(D) the risk of ovarian cancer is not related to marital status
(E) the risk of cancer of the testes is higher in married than in single men

191. When describing the epidemiology of lung cancer in the U.S. in 1990, all the following statements are true EXCEPT

(A) lung cancer is the leading cause of cancer death in men and women
(B) the 5-year survival rate from lung cancer is less than 20 percent
(C) more than 50 percent of patients have metastatic disease at the time of initial presentation
(D) the incidence of lung cancer in men is increasing
(E) the incidence of lung cancer in women is increasing

192. Cigarette smoking increases the risk of acquiring cancers of all the following EXCEPT

(A) esophagus
(B) pancreas
(C) larynx and oral cavity
(D) bladder and kidney
(E) liver

193. Multiple sclerosis (MS) is a chronic demyelinating disease characterized by an increased incidence in all the following EXCEPT

(A) women
(B) persons with certain HLA types
(C) persons who live in temperate rather than tropical climates
(D) blood relatives of persons with the disease
(E) blacks

194. All the following are associated with a poor prognosis in patients with pneumococcal pneumonia EXCEPT

(A) luekocytosis
(B) positive blood culture
(C) infection with type 3 pneumococcus
(D) patient's age less than 1 year
(E) meningitis

195. The most common site for cancer in persons in developing countries is

(A) cervix and uterus
(B) breast
(C) lung
(D) pharynx and oral cavity
(E) esophagus

196. The incidence of skin cancer

(A) is unaffected by environmental factors
(B) increases with age
(C) is higher in alcoholics
(D) is higher in persons who live far from the equator
(E) is higher in women

197. The reasons for the poor 5-year survival rate for pancreatic cancer include all the following EXCEPT

(A) the difficulty of establishing a diagnosis early during pathogenesis
(B) the usual ineffectiveness of radiotherapy
(C) the usual ineffectiveness of chemotherapy
(D) the unsuitability of about 85 percent of patients for resection at the time of diagnosis
(E) underlying diseases such as diabetes mellitus

198. Disorders of the prostate gland are a major cause of morbidity and mortality among elderly men. All the following statements about these disorders are true EXCEPT

(A) by age 80, almost 30 percent of men have benign prostatic hypertrophy
(B) about 10 percent of men will eventually undergo surgery for benign prostatic hypertrophy
(C) prostate cancer is the third most common cause of cancer death among men aged 56 and over in the U.S.
(D) prostate cancer is usually asymptomatic
(E) the incidence of prostate cancer is higher in blacks than in whites in the U.S.

199. All the following are associated with an increased risk of pulmonary thromboembolism EXCEPT

(A) hip fracture
(B) obesity
(C) surgery
(D) use of oral contraceptives
(E) hypertension

200. Although the etiology of adult rheumatoid arthritis is not known, studies of its epidemiology have shown that

(A) the incidence is 20 times higher in women than in men
(B) progressive joint destruction occurs in less than 20 percent of cases
(C) the vast majority of cases have their onset between the ages of 35 and 50
(D) there is no genetic predisposition to the disease
(E) there is an increased incidence of the disease in miners

201. True statements about osteoarthritis (degenerative joint disease) include

(A) it is more than twice as common among women as men of the same age
(B) the pattern of joint involvement is essentially identical in all races among persons of the same age
(C) osteoarthritis is the leading cause of disability in the elderly
(D) hereditary factors are important in Heberden's nodes
(E) none of the above

202. The probability that an asymptomatic person will suffer a stroke is increased with which of the following?

(A) A history of frequent headaches
(B) Alcoholism
(C) Electrocardiographic evidence of heart enlargement
(D) A type A personality
(E) None of the above

203. Factors associated with a poor prognosis in rheumatoid arthritis include all the following EXCEPT

(A) female sex
(B) high titers of rheumatoid factor
(C) subcutaneous nodules
(D) radiographic erosion on initial hand films
(E) symmetrical arthritis

204. The use of estrogen-containing oral contraceptives increases the risk of

(A) breast cancer
(B) vaginal cancer
(C) osteoporosis
(D) thromboembolism
(E) none of the above

205. Though much is still unknown about adult-onset diabetes mellitus, constitutional and environmental factors associated with an increased incidence of the disease include all the following EXCEPT

(A) obesity
(B) age
(C) family history of diabetes
(D) history of gestational diabetes
(E) high dietary sugar

206. Which of the following factors may contribute to development of chronic bronchitis?

(A) Use of nasal spray
(B) Altitude
(C) Occupation
(D) Alcohol abuse
(E) None of the above

207. Studies of the epidemiology of epilepsy have shown that

(A) brain tumor is the most common cause in children less than 12 years of age
(B) cerebrovascular disease is the most common cause in adults older than 50 years of age
(C) 20 to 25 percent of children will have one or more seizures with febrile illnesses at some time in their childhood
(D) 90 percent of patients with posttraumatic seizures require long-term anticonvulsant therapy
(E) seizures are more likely with rapidly growing malignancies, like glioblastomas

208. Complications of diabetes mellitus include all the following EXCEPT

(A) blindness
(B) pancreatic cancer
(C) limb loss
(D) myocardial infarction
(E) stroke

209. Epidemiologic investigations of testicular cancer have shown that

(A) the peak incidence occurs within 1 to 2 years of puberty
(B) there is an increased incidence in males with cryptorchidism
(C) there is an increased risk in males with a history of venereal disease
(D) there is an increased incidence in males with a family history of breast cancer
(E) there is no increased risk in males with a history of mumps orchitis

210. Exposure of nonsmokers to second-hand cigarette smoke may result in all the following EXCEPT

(A) increased incidence of osteoporosis
(B) elevation of blood concentration of carbon monoxide
(C) increased incidence of infections of the lower respiratory tract
(D) eye irritation, headache, nasal congestion, and cough
(E) exacerbation of chronic obstructive lung disease

211. Prognosis in Hodgkin's disease correlates with all the following EXCEPT

(A) the stage of disease at the time of diagnosis
(B) the presence of systemic symptoms
(C) the histologic type
(D) the sex of the patient
(E) HLA type

212. Factors that predispose males to testicular cancer include all the following EXCEPT

(A) inguinal hernia in childhood
(B) age of 20 to 35
(C) age over 50
(D) a history of mumps orchitis
(E) intraabdominal testicle

213. The incidence of ulcerative colitis in the U.S. is approximately 6 per 100,000 per year; the prevalence is about 100 per 100,000. The incidence of Crohn's disease in the U.S. is approximately 2 per 100,000 per year; the prevalence is about 30 per 100,000. The incidences of both diseases are higher in whites than in blacks, with an odds ratio of 2.0. Duration of the disease is similar in whites and blacks. This implies that in the U.S.

(A) the incidence of Crohn's disease in whites is about 5 per 100,000 per year
(B) the prevalence of ulcerative colitis in blacks is about 90 per 100,000
(C) the average duration of Crohn's disease is similar to that of ulcerative colitis
(D) the odds ratio is not a valid measure of the relative risk for these diseases
(E) there are approximately 15,000 persons in the U.S. with ulcerative colitis

214. Exposure to benzene has been associated with all the following diseases EXCEPT

(A) aplastic anemia
(B) bronchogenic carcinoma
(C) acute nonlymphocytic leukemia
(D) testicular atrophy
(E) chronic myelogenous leukemia

215. The development of neuropathic symptoms is associated with chronic exposure to all the following substances EXCEPT

(A) mercury
(B) lead
(C) arsenic
(D) sulfur dioxide
(E) nitrous oxide

216. Which of the following diseases is found almost exclusively among persons who have worked with or have been exposed to asbestos?

(A) Bronchogenic carcinoma
(B) Byssinosis
(C) Pleural mesothelioma
(D) Laryngeal carcinoma
(E) None of the above

217. Exposure to all of the following chemicals has been associated with kidney disease EXCEPT

(A) chlorine reaction products
(B) cadmium
(C) ethylene glycol
(D) halogenated hydrocarbons
(E) lead

218. Which one of the following is the major cause of skin cancer due to occupational exposure?

(A) Arsenic
(B) Coal tar
(C) Soot
(D) Radium and roentgen rays
(E) Ultraviolet light

219. Which of the following substances is causally associated with pneumoconiosis?

(A) Sulfur oxides
(B) Nitrogen oxides
(C) Oil fumes
(D) Dust particles
(E) Cigarette smoke

220. The most common asbestos-related tumor in humans is

(A) bronchogenic carcinoma
(B) carcinoma of the colon
(C) laryngeal carcinoma
(D) peritoneal mesothelioma
(E) pleural mesothelioma

221. Prolonged exposure to polyvinyl chlorides in production is associated with each of the following EXCEPT

(A) acroosteolysis
(B) Raynaud's syndrome
(C) lung disease
(D) angiosarcoma of the liver
(E) scleroderma-like skin changes

222. All the following statements about nonionizing radiation are true EXCEPT

(A) it includes radiowave and microwave frequencies
(B) its main adverse effects are related to cancer promotion and thermal injury
(C) excess exposure has been associated with an increased incidence of dermatologic neoplasms
(D) excess exposure has been associated with an increased incidence of cataracts
(E) excess exposure has been associated with an increased incidence of sterility

223. The industry that has the highest accidental death rate in the United States is

(A) manufacturing
(B) construction
(C) mining and quarrying
(D) transportation and public utilities
(E) service

224. Gout is a metabolic disease characterized by recurrent attacks of acute arthritis. Risk factors for gout include all the following EXCEPT

(A) hyperuricemia
(B) consumption of alcohol
(C) exposure to lead
(D) female gender
(E) use of diuretics

225. True statements about unintentional injuries in the U.S. include all the following EXCEPT

(A) injuries are the leading cause of death in children over 1 year of age
(B) motor vehicles account for almost one-third of deaths by unintentional injury in the U.S.
(C) deaths due to motor vehicle accidents are disproportionately high in adolescent males
(D) deaths due to falls are disproportionately high in the elderly
(E) about 1 person in 100 is hospitalized per year for injuries

226. Radiological findings specific for exposure to asbestos include

(A) bilateral pulmonary fibrosis
(B) pulmonary nodules
(C) pleural effusion
(D) pleural calcification
(E) none of the above

227. True statements about the epidemiology of sexually transmitted diseases (STDs) in the U.S. include

(A) persons aged 20 to 24 years are at highest risk for STDs
(B) for all age groups, homosexuals have a higher rate of STDs than do heterosexuals
(C) the frequent presence of cervical ectopy places adolescent females at higher risk of contracting *Neisseria gonorrhoeae* and *Chlamydia trachomatis*
(D) cervicitis is generally symptomatic
(E) none of the above

228. True statements about pneumoconiosis of coal workers (black lung) include which of the following?

(A) Progressive massive fibrosis occurs in more than half of coal workers who have pneumoconiosis
(B) Inhalation of anthracite (hard coal) dust is more dangerous than inhalation of bituminous (soft coal) dust
(C) Generally, large dust particles cause more scar formation than small dust particles
(D) It is not seen with silica-free coal dust
(E) None of the above

229. Exposure to methyl mercury (organic mercury) may cause all the following EXCEPT

(A) cerebral palsy
(B) paresthesias
(C) gingivitis
(D) coma
(E) visual deficits

230. The leading cause of end-stage renal disease (ESRD) in the U.S. is

(A) cystic kidney disease
(B) glomerulonephritis
(C) hypertension
(D) diabetes mellitus
(E) urinary tract obstruction

231. Workers associated with occupational exposure to lead include all the following EXCEPT

(A) battery makers
(B) producers of crystal glass
(C) coal miners
(D) solderers
(E) gasoline station attendants

232. Beta thalassemia is common in persons whose ancestors are from any of the following regions EXCEPT

(A) southern Italy
(B) central Africa
(C) Asia
(D) the Middle East
(E) Mediterranean islands

233. Loss of hearing due to exposure to noise depends upon all the following factors EXCEPT

(A) the duration of exposure
(B) the intensity of noise
(C) whether the noise is continuous or intermittent
(D) the frequency of the noise
(E) the atonality of the sound

234. Infectious agents of diarrheal diseases commonly encountered in patients with acquired immunodeficiency syndrome (AIDS) include all the following EXCEPT

(A) *Cryptosporidium*
(B) *Isospora belli*
(C) *Toxoplasma gondii*
(D) *Salmonella*
(E) cytomegalovirus

235. Syphilis has been increasing dramatically in the U.S. since the mid 1980s. True statements about congenital syphilis include all the following EXCEPT

(A) transmission can occur at any time during pregnancy
(B) penicillin is the treatment of choice
(C) tetracycline may be used in penicillin-sensitive mothers
(D) congenital infection may result in preterm delivery, low birth weight, or stillbirth
(E) manifestations of congenital syphilis range from asymptomatic disease to multisystem involvement

236. The most commonly described anomalies associated with congenital rubella include all the following EXCEPT

(A) cataracts
(B) sensorineural deafness
(C) microcephaly
(D) patent ductus arteriosus
(E) Hutchinson's teeth

237. True statements about lung diseases caused by inhalation of particles of crystalline silica include all the following EXCEPT

(A) they are some of the most common occupational lung diseases in the world
(B) they can be seen in persons with brief, intense exposures to silica dust
(C) chest radiographs may show small, rounded pulmonary nodules in the upper and middle lung fields
(D) a normal chest radiograph excludes the diagnosis of silicosis
(E) in industrialized countries cor pulmonale is the most frequent complication of silicosis

238. The most prevalent mental health disorder in young children is

(A) autism
(B) mental retardation
(C) behavioral problems
(D) schizophrenia
(E) depression

239. Epidemiological investigations of dementia in the U.S. have found all the following EXCEPT

(A) it is the major cause of long-term disability in old age
(B) 20 percent of persons above 80 years of age are afflicted
(C) AIDS encephalopathy is the most common cause of dementia
(D) that there is an increased incidence of Alzheimer's disease among relatives of patients with the disease
(E) dementia affects about 4 million people

240. Epidemiological studies of homosexuality have shown

(A) that the prevalence of homosexuality in the U.S. has increased in the past 20 years
(B) that homosexuality is five times as common among men as among women
(C) that the overall prevalence of homosexuality in the U. S. is about 1 percent
(D) that there is an increased incidence of homosexuality among relatives of male homosexuals
(E) none of the above

241. The most prevalent psychiatric disorder among opiate addicts undergoing treatment is

(A) schizophrenia
(B) depression
(C) alcoholism
(D) antisocial personality
(E) mania

242. Which of the following statements about the statistics of suicide is correct?

(A) Compared with other sex-race groups, the mortality from suicide is highest in black males of all ages
(B) The incidence of suicide attempts is higher in males than in females
(C) The risk of suicide increases for several months following divorce, separation, or death of the spouse
(D) Suicide rates do not correlate with socioeconomic status
(E) None of the above

243. True statements about the relationships between central nervous system damage and ingestion of lead include

(A) there are over 2 million children at risk in the U.S.
(B) effects on the central nervous system are reversible with chelating agents
(C) diagnosis of lead toxicity is complex
(D) lead does not pass across the placenta
(E) none of the above

244. What proportion of the United States population is estimated to have a mental or emotional problem that requires therapy?

(A) 1 percent
(B) 5 percent
(C) 10 percent
(D) 20 percent
(E) 40 percent

245. The psychosis most likely to occur in young adults (ages 15 to 24) is

(A) schizophrenia
(B) affective psychosis
(C) involutional melancholia
(D) agitated depression
(E) none of the above

246. In most states, the legal limit for blood alcohol concentration allowed while operating a motor vehicle is

(A) 50 mg/dL
(B) 100 mg/dL
(C) 200 mg/dL
(D) 300 mg/dL
(E) 400 mg/dL

247. Cancer is the fourth leading cause of death in U.S. adolescents aged 15 to 19. The leading cause of cancer death in this age group is

(A) lymphoma
(B) CNS tumors
(C) ovarian tumors
(D) bone tumors
(E) leukemia

248. Which of the following statements about alcoholism is true?

(A) There are about 30 million alcoholics in the U.S.
(B) About 10 percent of the population consumes 95 percent of the alcohol
(C) The incidence of alcoholism is highest among college graduates
(D) The incidence of alcoholism is about the same in men and women
(E) None of the above

249. Studies of the epidemiology of alcoholism have shown

(A) that it is often associated with a family history of strict abstinence
(B) that there is only weak evidence for a genetic cause
(C) that the usual age of onset in men is about age 40, during the midlife crisis
(D) that there is a secondary peak in incidence after age 65
(E) none of the above

250. Which statement best represents a correct and generally accepted finding obtained in current epidemiologic studies of autistic children?

(A) Autistic children are most often members of lower socioeconomic families
(B) Autistic children are most often members of higher socioeconomic families
(C) Parents of autistic children are often emotionally frigid and introverted
(D) Autism is more prevalent among boys than girls
(E) Autism does not have a genetic cause

251. Which of the following persons is most likely to commit suicide?

(A) A 65-year-old widower
(B) A 40-year-old married father
(C) A 30-year-old unmarried woman
(D) A 30-year-old divorced man
(E) A 16-year-old girl

252. Which of the following statements best describes the incidence of suicide?

(A) The peak incidence of suicide occurs in persons who are in their early twenties and then the incidence declines

(B) The peak incidence of suicide occurs in middle-aged persons and then the incidence declines

(C) The incidence of suicide increases directly with age

(D) The incidence of suicide decreases directly with age

(E) the incidence of suicide is equal at all ages

253. Which of the following statements about the relationship between religion and suicide in the U.S. is true?

(A) There is no relationship between religion and suicide

(B) Catholics are at a higher risk of suicide than Protestants

(C) Catholics are at a higher risk of suicide than Jews

(D) Religious people are at a higher risk of suicide than those who are not religious

(E) None of the above

254. Persons with sickle cell disease are at increased risk for fulminant infections by all the following EXCEPT

(A) *Neisseria meningitidis*
(B) *Streptococcus pneumoniae*
(C) *Plasmodium malariae*
(D) *Babesia microti*
(E) *Chlamydia trachomatis*

255. True statements about social determinants of health include all the following EXCEPT

(A) divorced persons have greater mortality from cancer than do married persons

(B) persons with few social ties (friends, activities) have greater mortality from coronary heart disease than do persons with many social ties

(C) persons of lower socioeconomic status have greater mortality from diabetes than do persons of higher socioeconomic status

(D) after correcting for race and access to medical care, there is still a relationship between socioeconomic status and mortality

(E) female sex is associated with increased mortality from most diseases

256. Chronic barbiturate abuse is particularly common among

(A) unemployed teenagers
(B) college students
(C) middle-aged women
(D) elderly women
(E) elderly men

257. Which of the following mental disorders has its highest incidence in the geriatric population?

(A) Involutional depression
(B) Anxiety disorder
(C) Obsessive-compulsive disorder
(D) Schizophrenia
(E) None of the above

258. Which of the following features characterizes families in which spouse abuse occurs?

(A) Husbands of battered women are frequently substance abusers
(B) Women who were abused as children are more likely to be abused as adults
(C) Women whose mothers suffered abuse are unlikely to be abused by their own husbands
(D) Men who batter women are prosecuted in 25 percent of cases
(E) None of the above

259. The incidence of anorexia nervosa has been increasing recently. True statements about this disease include

(A) it is two to three times more common in females than males
(B) there is an increased incidence in the middle and upper classes
(C) it usually involves a profound loss of appetite in its early stages
(D) its usual age of onset is in the twenties or thirties
(E) none of the above

260. The mental disorders that appear to be more prevalent among males include

(A) alcoholism and drug abuse
(B) schizophrenia
(C) neuroses
(D) affective disorders
(E) none of the above

261. Panic disorders are characterized by the sudden onset of overwhelming terror or anxiety. True statements about the incidence of panic disorders include which of the following?

(A) They are twice as common in women as in men
(B) The usual age of onset is less than 15 years of age
(C) There is an increased incidence in family members of index patients
(D) They affect about 1 in 1000 persons
(E) None of the above

262. Which of the following statements correctly describes emotional disturbances of the postpartum period?

(A) They are more common after the birth of male children

(B) They are more common with increasing parity

(C) They rarely last more than 1 week

(D) They occur in at least 20 percent of women

(E) None of the above

263. Parents who abuse their children are correctly characterized by all the following statements EXCEPT

(A) they are more likely to be alcoholics than are nonabusive parents

(B) they are found in all social classes

(C) they are more likely to have been abused as children than are nonabusive parents

(D) they are more likely to be men than women

(E) they are usually psychologically immature

264. True statements about the use of opioid drugs in the U.S. include

(A) the highest rates of use occur among persons 30 to 40 years of age

(B) more men than women use opioid drugs other than heroin

(C) the number of male users of heroin is 50 percent greater than the number of female users

(D) less than 1 percent of enlisted personnel in the military use opioid drugs

(E) none of the above

265. Stuttering is a disturbance of the normal speech rhythm and fluency and is characterized by

(A) an increased incidence in girls compared with boys

(B) an increased incidence among family members of stutterers

(C) an increased incidence in whites compared with non-whites

(D) a peak incidence among adolescents

(E) none of the above

266. Studies of attempted (unsuccessful) suicide have shown which of the following?

(A) It is 100 times more common than completed (successful) suicide
(B) About 10 percent of persons who attempt suicide eventually commit suicide
(C) It is most common in persons with obsessive-compulsive personalities
(D) It is more common among women than men
(E) None of the above

267. Population-based epidemiologic surveys in the U.S. using standardized diagnostic interviews have been conducted among adults ages 18 and over. According to the responses to these surveys, which of the following statements is true?

(A) Alcohol abuse or dependence is the most prevalent mental disorder among men over age 65
(B) About one person in twenty has been affected by a significant mental disorder within the previous 6 months
(C) Most persons affected by a mental disorder are receiving some sort of psychiatric care
(D) Phobias are the most prevalent mental disorder in women of all ages
(E) None of the above

268. Persons at increased risk of bladder cancer include all the following EXCEPT

(A) workers in the rubber industry
(B) workers who handle textile dyes
(C) workers in the steel industry
(D) persons with chronic *Schistosoma haematobium* infection
(E) cigarette smoker

269. There are approximately 7500 new cases of Hodgkin's disease annually in the U.S. Epidemiological studies show risk factors for the development of Hodgkin's disease include all the following EXCEPT

(A) immunodeficiency disease
(B) infection with Epstein-Barr virus
(C) male sex
(D) age 15 to 35 years
(E) age over 50 years

270. Risk factors associated with the development of osteoporosis include all the following EXCEPT

(A) excessive alcohol intake
(B) obesity
(C) white race
(D) poor calcium intake during adolescence
(E) postmenopausal state

271. Occupational activities associated with preterm delivery include all the following EXCEPT

(A) work extending beyond 40 h per week
(B) prolonged standing (> 4 h at one time)
(C) repetitive heavy lifting
(D) night-shift work
(E) third-trimester employment

272. All the following are true statements about tuberculosis EXCEPT

(A) humans are the only reservoir of *Mycobacterium tuberculosis*
(B) the causative agents of human tuberculosis include *M. bovis*
(C) the primary infection is often asymptomatic
(D) the time from infection to the development of a positive tuberculin skin test averages 6 months
(E) HIV infection is an independent risk factor for the development of active tuberculosis

273. True statements about teenage (15 to 19 years old) pregnancy in the U.S. include all the following EXCEPT

(A) approximately 1 in 9 teenagers becomes pregnant each year
(B) greater than three-fourths of these pregnancies are unintended
(C) 10 percent of births to teens are repeat births
(D) approximately 40 percent of all teen pregnancies are aborted
(E) one-fifth of premarital teen pregnancies occur within the first month of commencing intercourse

DIRECTIONS: Each group of questions below consists of lettered headings followed by a set of numbered items. For each numbered item select the **one** lettered heading with which it is **most** closely associated. Each lettered heading may be used **once, more than once, or not at all.**

Questions 274–277

Match each of the diseases below with the pattern of occurrence in day-care centers.

(A) Infection affects children in day care, day-care center staff, and close family members
(B) Infection is generally unapparent in the children, but symptomatic in adult contacts
(C) Infection is mild in children in day care and in adult contacts, but may cause significant disease in the fetus if pregnant women are exposed
(D) Infection does not occur at an increased rate in day-care centers
(E) None of the above

274. Hepatitis A

275. Cytomegalovirus

276. Giardiasis

277. Leptospirosis

Questions 278–280

For each disease or condition, select the best available source of information.

(A) Death certificates
(B) Household surveys
(C) Cancer registry
(D) State health department
(E) Life insurance companies

278. Incidence of meningococcal meningitis in Connecticut

279. Prevalence of arthritis

280. Survival rate of patients with cancer of the pancreas

Questions 281–284

Match each group of diseases with the correct description.

(A) Bacterial infections
(B) Zoonoses
(C) Person-to-person spread
(D) Viral infections
(E) Arthropod-borne infections

281. Rabies, psittacosis, salmonellosis

282. Influenza, yellow fever, chickenpox

283. Pneumococcal, streptococcal, brucellar infections

284. Measles, shigellosis, scabies

Questions 285–288

Various terms and parameters are used in epidemiological studies of infectious diseases. Match each statement below with the most appropriate descriptive term.

(A) Immunogenicity
(B) Pathogenicity
(C) Contagiousness
(D) Virulence
(E) None of the above

285. Neutralizing antibody develops in 95 percent of people after an attack of measles

286. Febrile respiratory tract disease develops in approximately 80 percent of children infected with influenza

287. Death occurs in approximately 20 percent of cases of pneumococcal meningitis

288. Approximately 50 percent of household contacts of a child who has a common cold become infected

Questions 289–292

Choose the most likely infectious agent for each description of the events following consumption of food.

(A) Staphylococcal enterotoxin
(B) *Clostridium botulinum* toxin
(C) Enterotoxic *Escherichia coli*
(D) *Clostridium perfringens*
(E) *Salmonella typhimurium*

289. Within 4 h after attending a church supper, 25 persons report the abrupt onset of nausea, vomiting, and abdominal cramps

290. One week after arriving in Africa, 16 students develop vomiting, severe diarrhea, and abdominal cramps lasting 2 to 3 days

291. A patient dies of respiratory failure after an illness characterized by weakness, diplopia, and cranial nerve paresis

292. One-third of the persons who attended a school banquet develop abdominal cramps and watery diarrhea 8 to 12 h later. These symptoms end within 24 h

Questions 293–296

Match each of the descriptions below with the correct type of arthritis.

(A) Gout
(B) Rheumatoid arthritis
(C) Osteoarthritis
(D) Sarcoid arthritis
(E) None of the above

293. It is often iatrogenic

294. It usually begins in childhood

295. It is the most common form of arthritis in the southeastern U.S.

296. One subtype is associated with HLA-DR4

Questions 297–300

Match each of the chronic diseases below with the virus with which it has been most closely associated.

(A) Hepatitis A virus (HAV)
(B) Hepatitis B virus (HBV)
(C) Hepatitis E virus (HEV)
(D) Varicella-zoster virus (VZV)
(E) Epstein-Barr virus (EBV)

297. Nasopharyngeal carcinoma

298. Hepatoma

299. Burkitt's lymphoma

300. Polyarteritis nodosa

Questions 301–305

Many occupational environments contain airborne substances that cause lung disease. For each disease, select the worker with whom it is associated.

(A) Hay farmer
(B) Radar assembly worker
(C) Arc welder
(D) Coal worker
(E) Textile worker

301. Berylliosis

302. Hypersensitivity pneumonitis

303. Byssinosis

304. Caplan's syndrome

305. Siderosis

Questions 306–310

Match each of the workers or hobbyists below with the infectious disease for which they are at risk.

(A) Brucellosis
(B) Hepatitis B
(C) Histoplasmosis
(D) Legionnaires' disease
(E) Sporotrichosis

306. Butchers

307. Gardners

308. Air-conditioning workers

309. Dentists

310. Spelunkers (cave explorers)

Questions 311–315

Match each of the workers below with the factor that constitutes the principal hazard to health.

(A) Silica dust
(B) Carbon monoxide
(C) Vinyl acetate
(D) Hydrogen sulfide
(E) Asbestos

311. Brake mechanic

312. Potter

313. Glass manufacturer

314. Sewer worker

315. Arc welder

Questions 316–319

For each of the age groups below, select the most common cause of death.

(A) Heart disease
(B) Cancer
(C) Stroke
(D) Pneumonia
(E) Automobile crashes

316. 1 to 14 years

317. 15 to 24 years

318. 25 to 44 years

319. 45 to 64 years

Questions 320–324

Certain substances in the occupational environment have been identified as carcinogenic agents based on epidemiological evidence obtained in studies of exposed laboratory animal and human populations. Match each chemical agent with the human target site for cancer.

(A) Liver
(B) Brain
(C) Bladder
(D) Lung
(E) Hematopoietic system

320. β-Naphthylamine (amino-naphthalene)

321. Benzene (benzol)

322. Nickel

323. Chromium

324. Asbestos

DIRECTIONS: The group of questions below consists of four lettered headings followed by a set of numbered items. For each numbered item select

A	if the item is associated with	(A) **only**
B	if the item is associated with	(B) **only**
C	if the item is associated with	**both** (A) and (B)
D	if the item is associated with	**neither** (A) nor (B)

Each lettered heading may be used **once, more than once, or not at all.**

Questions 325–328

   (A) Tobacco
   (B) Alcohol
   (C) Both
   (D) Neither

325. Esophageal cancer

326. Cervical cancer

327. Duodenal ulcer

328. Hip fracture

Epidemiology of Health and Disease

Answers

131. The answer is B. *(Wilson, 12/e, pp 1016–1017.)* Hypertension, not hypercholesterolemia, is the major risk factor for aortic dissection. Several diseases of connective tissue—including Marfan's syndrome, Hurler's disease, and cystic medial necrosis—are associated with an increased incidence of aortic dissection. Operative mortality is about 50 percent for emergency surgery for ascending aortic dissection. Acute dissection usually presents with chest pain, classically a tearing pain that radiates to the back.

132. The answer is C. *(Last, Maxcy-Rosenau, 13/e, pp 203–207.)* Five to ten percent of patients admitted to general hospitals in the United States acquire an infection while in the hospital. University and municipal hospitals generally have higher rates of nosocomial infections than small community hospitals. The incidence is two to three times higher in chronic-disease hospitals compared with acute-care institutions.

133. The answer is E. *(Mausner, 2/e, pp 344–345.)* The most important risk factor for breast cancer (like most cancers) is age: the rate in women 75 to 84 years old is about 50 times that of women 35 to 44 years old. If crude incidence rates are compared (new cases per 100,000 adult women), one country may have much larger numbers of women in the peak risk groups and have a much higher incidence for that reason. Therefore, either comparison of the age-specific rates for each age group or else some type of *age adjustment* is essential. Although nursing may have a protective effect on breast cancer, it is of nowhere near the magnitude of the effect of age. Cigarette smoke is not a major risk factor for breast cancer. Early diagnosis, if it had any effect, would be expected to increase the incidence rate (since some cases might be discovered that otherwise might spontaneously resolve or not be noticed before the woman died of another cause). Finally, efficacy of treatment might affect the death rate, but would not affect the incidence of the disease.

134. The answer is E. *(Wilson, 12/e, pp 1298–1299.)* Appendicitis remains an important cause of morbidity in the Western world. Although its incidence is increasing, the mortality is decreasing. Boys and girls are about equally affected (with perhaps a 3:2 ratio of boys to girls). It is most common in the second and third decades of life. During pregnancy, displacement of the appendix by the gravid uterus can make diagnosis difficult.

135. The answer is B. *(Last, Maxcy-Rosenau, 13/e, pp 43, 1115.)* Infant mortality is defined as the number of deaths in infants less than 1 year of age per 1000 *live* births for a given year. It is further divided into neonatal mortality, which includes deaths up to 28 days of age, and postneonatal mortality, which includes deaths from 28 days to 1 year of age. In the U.S., about two-thirds of infant mortality occurs in the first 28 days of life, and the most important cause is prematurity. The most important cause of postneonatal mortality is the sudden infant death syndrome (SIDS). American blacks have twice the rates of low birth weight, neonatal mortality, and postneonatal mortality of whites.

136. The answer is E. *(Wilson, 12/e, pp 1298–1299.)* Perforation of the appendix, with subsequent peritonitis, is the main complication of appendicitis. Up to 80 percent of infants with appendicitis will have perforated appendices at the time of presentation. Surgical mortality is 30 times higher in the presence of perforation.

137. The answer is E. *(Benenson, 15/e, pp 83–86.)* The major problems associated with chickenpox are its significant morbidity in children, including its association with Reye syndrome and the administration of aspirin; the reactivation of the virus as herpes zoster in later life; and the high morbidity and mortality in immunosuppressed patients. The case fatality rate of chickenpox in normal children is very low. Malformations from gestational chickenpox exposure are very rare (*rubella* is the disease for which this is the major concern). Infection generally confers lifelong immunity, so reinfection is rare. The *incubation* period during which time the patient is asymptomatic is up to 3 weeks, but the *prodromal* period (of mild symptoms) is short.

138. The answer is D. *(Benenson, 15/e, pp 182–185.)* Giardiasis occurs all over the world, and epidemics resulting from contamination of water supplies by the protozoan *Giardia lamblia* have occurred in Russia and the United States. Giardiasis is usually a noninvasive infection of the small intestine and has a spectrum of illness ranging from asymptomatic carriage to severe chronic diarrhea. Unlike *Entamoeba histolytica,* the cause of amebiasis, *G. lamblia* does not invade the colonic mucosa. Person-to-person transmission is frequent in day-care centers.

139. The answer is E. *(Rudolph, 18/e, p 567.)* For every infant with classic symptoms of CMV infection—including microcephaly, chorioretinitis, deafness, hepatosplenomegaly, jaundice, and thrombocytopenia—there are probably 20 infants without symptoms. Neurological sequelae of intrauterine exposure to CMV include mental retardation, minimal cerebral dysfunction, and sensorineural hearing loss. The prevalence of infection at birth is as high as 2.5 percent in some communities.

140. The answer is B. *(Wilson, 12/e, p 1048.)* Boys develop asthma about twice as commonly as girls. Childhood asthma tends to be more allergic. There are higher levels of IgE in the serum, more frequent positive responses to inhaled antigens, and seasonal variations.

141. The answer is C. *(Rudolph, 18/e, pp 485, 1696.)* The most common causes (in decreasing order of incidence) of bacterial meningitis in children 3 months to 6 years of age are *Haemophilus influenzae* type b, *Neisseria meningitidis,* and *Streptococcus pneumoniae.* The latter two bacteria cause most cases of meningitis in adults. *Escherichia coli* K1 and group B *Streptococcus* are the most common causes of neonatal meningitis.

142. The answer is E. *(Wilson, 12/e, p 469.)* Transmission of bacteria from patient to patient most often occurs via the hands of hospital personnel. Airborne transmission, indirect exposure, and common-source exposure do occur but are much less important than direct spread. Indwelling catheters are an important risk factor for nosocomial infections but are not sources of transmission of infections.

143. The answer is D. *(Wilson, 12/e, pp 1041–1053.)* Acute episodes of asthma have been associated with a wide variety of triggers, including dust, animal dander, respiratory infections, ozone pollution, aspirin, and emotional factors. Asthma is an episodic disease of the airways characterized by increased responsiveness of the tracheobronchial tree to these and other stimuli. There are allergic and idiosyncratic forms of asthma. Caffeine is a methylxanthine related to theophylline and is a low-potency bronchodilator.

144. The answer is D. *(Last, Maxcy-Rosenau, 13/e, pp 1021–1027.)* Injuries are the leading cause of death in the younger members of the U.S. population. Motor vehicle accidents, drowning, and fire-related injuries account for the majority of these deaths.

145. The answer is D. *(Last, Maxcy-Rosenau, 13/e, pp 203–207.)* Urinary tract infections (UTIs) are the most common hospital-acquired infection and account for 35 percent of all nosocomial infections. Approximately 70 to 80 percent of nosocomial UTIs are related to urinary catheters or urinary tract manipulation. Infections of surgical wounds are the second most common nosocomial infection, followed by infections of the lower respiratory tract and blood stream.

146. The answer is B. *(Last, Maxcy-Rosenau, 13/e, pp 1035–1038.)* Each year more than 20,000 people die from homicide in the United States. Homicide is the third leading cause of death for persons aged 15 to 24 years and the leading cause of death for black males aged 15 to 34 years. Approximately 20 percent of homicides are committed during the perpetration of another felony or crime; 55 percent of U.S. homicides involve friends, acquaintances, or family members. The lifetime risk of death from homicide for white U.S. males is 1 in 64; it is 1 in 28 for black males.

147. The answer is C. *(Wilson, 12/e, pp 1327–1328.)* Most cases of posttransfusion hepatitis are due to hepatitis C virus; until recently, there was no way to screen for this virus. The risk is highest for products, such as individual clotting factors, obtained from multiple pooled donors. Albumin and immune globulin convey no risk because these products receive special treatments. Hepatitis C can be a serious illness and progress to chronic hepatitis in about half of cases.

148. The answer is D. *(Last, Maxcy-Rosenau, 13/e, pp 834–836.)* Obesity is a major risk factor for non-insulin-dependent diabetes, but it is relatively unimportant as a risk factor for coronary heart disease except at extremes of the weight distribution. Over the last 20 years dramatic declines in U.S. deaths due to cardiovascular disease (CVD), despite the clearly increasing average U.S. body mass, indicate that risk factors other than obesity are of primary importance in the development of cardiovascular disease. Obesity is commonly considered to be present when body fat exceeds 25 percent of body weight in men and 30 percent of body weight in women. Both behavioral and genetic factors contribute to obesity.

149. The answer is E. *(Wilson, 12/e, pp 1576–1577.)* Cancer is the second leading cause of death in the U.S. (after heart disease). About 500,000 Americans die annually from cancer, almost one-third from lung cancer. Nonmelanomatous skin cancers are the most common cancer, and lung cancer is the most common cause of cancer mortality in the U.S.

150. The answer is C. *(Last, Maxcy-Rosenau, 13/e, pp 1006–1007.)* The decayed, missing, or filled (DMF) rate is the average number of teeth per person that are identified as decayed, missing, or filled. The DMF rate is used to determine the prevalence of caries. The calculus index and the oral hygiene index measure the amount of plaque and debris formation. These indices are indirectly related to dental caries since plaque formation precedes the development of caries. The malocclusion index is a measure of the need for orthodontic care and is therefore unrelated to dental caries.

151. The answer is B. *(Rudolph, 18/e, pp 540, 577.)* Outbreaks of fever, pharyngitis, and conjunctivitis have been linked to transmission of adenovirus in swimming pools. Although the effects of penicillin on the course of pharyngitis have been debated for some time, it is now clear that resolution is hastened by penicillin, at least in children. Although rhinoviruses can be transmitted before the onset of symptoms, patients are most infectious when the symptoms are the worst. Numerous viruses, including adenovirus, herpes simplex, influenza, and parainfluenza viruses can cause sore throats, but the most common identifiable pathogen is easily the group A streptococcus, which accounts for about a third of cases.

152. The answer is D. *(Wilson, 12/e, pp 969–970.)* There is wide variation in mortality for coronary artery bypass surgery performed by different surgeons and hospitals, and this variation cannot be explained simply by differences in severity of disease. Operative mortality is also higher among the elderly. Perioperative myocardial infarction occurs in about 5 to 10 percent of patients; usually, the infarcts are small.

153. The answer is C. *(Wilson, 12/e, pp 411–417.)* Arthritis, particularly of the hip, is more common in obese subjects, probably because of mechanical stresses on the joints. Recent studies have shown that it is not only the number of calories consumed but their composition that determines weight gain. Normal subjects can compensate for excessive carbohydrate intake by increasing their metabolic rate. Obese subjects are less active than normal subjects, but the inactivity is probably at least partially a result, rather than a cause, of the obesity. The association between hypertension and obesity is real; it is not a result of inappropriate cuff size.

154. The answer is D. *(Rudolph, 18/e, pp 158–159, 1019–1021.)* Colostrum and mature breast milk contain significant amounts of immunoglobulins, especially secretory IgA. The immunoglobulins, along with other resistance factors such as maternal macrophages, contribute to the lower incidence of infections in breast-fed compared with bottle-fed infants. Infants absorb more iron from human than from bovine milk. Cow's milk may also lead to iron deficiency by causing occult gastrointestinal blood loss.

155. The answer is D. *(Wilson, 12/e, p 1613.)* First-degree relatives (siblings, parents, and children) have a two- to threefold increased risk of developing breast cancer compared with the general population. The lifetime risk for developing breast cancer in the United States is 1 in 8.

156. The answer is C. *(Wilson, 12/e, pp 965, 995–996.)* Coronary heart disease (CHD) is synonymous with ischemic heart disease and arteriosclerotic heart disease. In the U.S., CHD is the leading cause of death in men by age 35 and women by age 45. Males constitute approximately 80 percent of all patients with angina pectoris, which is an episodic clinical syndrome due to transient myocardial ischemia.

157. The answer is D. *(Last, Maxcy-Rosenau, 13/e, pp 811–822.)* Colon cancer accounts for about 10 percent of all cancer deaths in the U.S. It is the second leading cause of cancer death in men (after lung cancer) and the third leading cause of cancer death in women (after lung and breast cancer). The exact etiology is unknown, but low-fat diets and those high in fiber are inversely associated with risk for colon cancer. Genetics may play a role; for example, persons with untreated familial polyposis generally develop colon cancer. Alcohol and tobacco have not consistently been associated with colon cancer.

158. The answer is A. *(Wilson, 12/e, pp 1019–1020.)* The majority of patients with peripheral vascular disease (the usual cause of intermittent claudication) also have coronary artery disease; the opposite is not true. The most powerful risk factor for the development of peripheral vascular disease is cigarette smoking. Only about 5 percent of patients with intermittent claudication eventually require amputation.

159. The answer is A. *(Wilson, 12/e, pp 1249–1250.)* The incidence of gastric cancer in men is twice that in women. Gastric cancer is common in Japan, Chile, and China; it is much less common in the United States. The steady decline in the incidence of gastric cancer over the past 40 years has not been adequately explained. Japanese people who have migrated to the United States continue to have a high incidence, but the incidence in their offspring is similar to the overall incidence of persons in the United States. These data are evidence of an environmental etiologic factor in the disease. Smokers and patients with benign gastric ulcers are not at increased risk.

160. The answer is E. *(Wyngaarden, 18/e, p 35.)* Because they affect young people disproportionately, injuries are the most important cause of premature loss of life in the U.S. Cancer, which also has a relatively high incidence among the young, is second. Coronary disease, the most important overall cause of death, mainly affects older persons. Congenital heart disease is too rare to be an important cause of premature loss of life. In some communities, AIDS is now the leading cause of premature loss of life.

161. The answer is E. *(Last, Maxcy-Rosenau, 13/e, pp 937–944.)* Chronic infection of the tarsal conjunctiva with *Chlamydia trachomatis* causes blindness by scarring of the conjunctiva and eventual opacification of the exposed cornea, not by predisposing to retinal detachment. The poorer the hygiene, the greater the chance for reinfection. Thus trachoma is the leading cause of blindness among persons who live in dry environments without access to sufficient water for washing. Cataracts are also a common cause of blindness in the world because of inadequate access to surgical facilities. In the U.S., the leading cause of blindness among whites is retinal disease, especially age-related macular degeneration; among blacks, glaucoma is the most important (and preventable) cause. Persons with high degrees of myopia (nearsightedness) have elongated eyes with retinas that are susceptible to detachment. Type I (and, to a lesser extent, type II) diabetics are at risk for proliferative retinopathy. In this condition, new blood vessels form on the retina; these vessels are fragile and may cause vitreous hemorrhage and retinal detachment.

162. The answer is D. *(Wilson, 12/e, p 1526.)* Cobalamin deficiency can be caused by a variety of conditions. The most common cause in temperate climates is pernicious anemia, in which the gastric mucosa is atrophied due to an autoimmune reaction against gastric parietal cells.

There is also an increased incidence in patients with a personal or family history of autoimmune diseases, such as Graves' disease. Destruction of gastric parietal cells following injury may also result in cobalamin deficiency, as can infection with the fish tapeworm *Diphyllobothrium latum*. Although cobalamin deficiency is found with tropical sprue, it is rarely a complication of nontropical sprue.

163. The answer is B. *(Wilson, 12/e, pp 1520–1521.)* The most common causes of microcytic anemia in the U.S. are iron deficiency, lead poisoning, thalassemia, and the anemia of chronic disease. Iron deficiency on a dietary basis is the most common cause in children and menstruating or pregnant women. However, iron deficiency is rarely seen on a dietary basis in men; finding it mandates a search for a (gastrointestinal) site of blood loss. Pica (a desire to eat unusual substances) can be associated with anemia. Infection with hookworms, but not pinworms, is an important worldwide cause of iron-deficiency anemia.

164. The answer is A. *(Wilson, 12/e, p 1293.)* Prognosis in colon cancer depends upon a variety of factors, including some related to the characteristics of the cancer cells. Tumors with aneuploid cells have higher rates of metastasis. When adjusted for nodal involvement and histologic differentiation, tumor size is not an independent predictor of poor outcome.

165. The answer is C. *(Last, 13/e, p 873.)* The prevalence of diabetes increases substantially with age, and most elderly diabetics have type II diabetes. About 2 percent of all Americans have diabetes; of those over age 70 years, the prevalence is about 10 percent. Because type II diabetes can be relatively asymptomatic, up to half of all diabetics may be undiagnosed.

166. The answer is A. *(Wilson, 12/e, p 1437.)* Rheumatoid arthritis afflicts women three times more than men. Its highest incidence is in the fourth and fifth decades of life. Differences in race, geographic residence, and social, economic, or cultural characteristics have not been related to the prevalence of this systemic disease of unknown cause.

167. The answer is B. *(Wilson, 12/e, p 1289.)* Evidence from international studies suggests that colon cancer rates are high in countries in which average consumption of animal fats is high. Several conditions associated with chronic inflammation of the colon—including Crohn's disease, ulcerative colitis, and the presence of a ureterosigmoidostomy—also predispose to colon cancer. Additional risk factors may include diets low in dietary fiber.

168. The answer is D. *(Wilson, 12/e, pp 933–946.)* Rheumatic heart disease is a major problem in many developing countries, and in the past several years, local outbreaks have occurred in the U.S. Persons with a history of rheumatic fever are at a substantially increased risk of recurrence, and prophylactic therapy (such as monthly injections of benzathine penicillin) is recommended. Coronary artery disease does not cause valvular heart disease. A myocardial infarction may cause mitral regurgitation with a normal valve because of papillary muscle necrosis. Echocardiographic surveys have found that up to 7 percent of women between the ages of 14 and 30 have mitral valve prolapse; most are asymptomatic.

169. The answer is D. *(Last, Maxcy-Rosenau, 13/e, pp 886–887. Wilson, 12/e, pp 1072–1074.)* Cystic fibrosis is the most common *semilethal* genetic disease in whites in the U.S. The incidence is about 1 in 2000 live births; about 5 percent of the white population are carriers of the gene (heterozygotes). It is a multisystem disorder characterized by abnormal exocrine gland function. The diagnosis can be confirmed by finding elevated levels of chloride (> 70 meq/L) in the sweat.

170. The answer is D. *(Wilson, 12/e, pp 1047–1053.)* Asthma is characterized by reversible bronchospasm. Between episodes FEV_1 may be entirely normal. Its cause is unknown but may be related to intrinsic (stress) or extrinsic (allergenic) factors. Almost 20 percent of patients have their first attack *after* age 40. Although the disease is more frequent in boys than girls, the sex difference disappears in adulthood.

171. The answer is B. *(Wilson, 12/e, p 1072.)* Cystic fibrosis is the most common semilethal genetic disorder in white Americans; nearly 1 in 20 carries the gene. Median survival is now about 20 years. Nearly all (98 percent) men with cystic fibrosis are infertile. DNA probes allow prenatal diagnosis and carrier detection.

172. The answer is C. *(Wilson, 12/e, pp 1074–1078.)* The accepted diagnosis of emphysema requires examination of lung tissue. Along with chronic bronchitis, emphysema causes chronic (irreversible) obstructive airways disease. The two diseases cause decreased expiratory flow rates. Heavy smokers are more likely to develop emphysema than light smokers. Inhalation of coal dust is associated with pneumoconiosis, a form of restrictive lung disease. Clinicopathologic correlations show that the majority of adults with emphysema are asymptomatic.

173. The answer is B. *(Wilson, 12/e, pp 1792–1793.)* Among women ages 40 to 44, the highest mortality occurs among those using birth control pills, especially among smokers. In general, the mortality risk of birth control pills is about five times higher in smokers. Mortality in IUD users is similar at all ages. The highest birth-related death rates (about 28 per 100,000 women per year) occur in women ages 40 to 44; this compares with a mortality of 1.5 per 100,000 women of all ages associated with abortions.

174. The answer is E. *(Last, Maxcy-Rosenau, 13/e, pp 1277–1279.)* Disorders of the musculoskeletal system are the most common cause of limitation of activity in the U.S. They affect about 12 million persons (about 8 million persons are affected by cardiovascular disease, the second leading cause). Back and spine impairments, which are the most common type, account for about half of these cases. Persons who engage in heavy labor, especially if it involves lifting and stooping, are more likely to have back pain than are sedentary workers. X-rays and medical examinations are not reliable ways to identify persons at high risk of sustaining a back injury; strength testing seems to be a better method.

175. The answer is B. *(Wilson, 12/e, pp 1069–1070.)* Bronchiectasis is quite common in childhood and either may begin as an infection of the bronchi and bronchioles that causes necrosis or may be the consequence of some abnormal physiological mechanism that causes abnormal dilatation, poor drainage, and secondary infection. Cough, fever, and production of copious amounts of malodorous sputum are characteristic symptoms of bronchiectasis, which can affect persons of any age or sex. Bronchiectasis may persist as a chronic, smoldering, latent infection.

176. The answer is E. *(Wilson, 12/e, p 312.)* Cutaneous reactions are one of the most frequent adverse reactions to drugs. Penicillins, sulfonamides, and blood products account for two-thirds of all cutaneous reactions. Exanthems are the most common skin manifestation. Cutaneous drug reactions usually occur within 1 week of drug exposure; reactions to semisynthetic penicillins and ampicillin, however, may present 2 to 4 weeks following initial exposure. The incidence of cutaneous drug reactions is higher in women but not the elderly.

177. The answer is E. *(Last, Maxcy-Rosenau, 13/e, pp 827–829.)* The death rate due to coronary artery disease (CAD) varies from country to country, from a low of about 275 per 100,000 men aged 35 to 74 years in Japan to a high of nearly 1000 per 100,000 men in Finland. Most areas of Europe have higher rates than the U.S. Finland has the highest death rate due to CAD in the world; this is perhaps related to a high per capita consumption of animal fat. The low rate of CAD in Japan is thought to be related to diet. The death rate due to CAD in the U.S. has been declining. This trend is associated with changes in medical care as well as changes in the population distribution of risk factors.

178. The answer is B. *(Last, Maxcy-Rosenau, 13/e, p 933.)* Hypertension is the major risk factor for strokes, and treatment of high blood pressure is the most efficacious way to prevent stroke. Other risk factors for strokes include smoking, vascular disease, transient ischemic attacks, and diabetes mellitus.

179. The answer is D. *(Wilson, 12/e, p 16.)* Most of the differences in life expectancy between men and women are primarily a result of lower rates of smoking, drinking of alcohol, and violent deaths in women. Nearly three times as many elderly women as men live alone; women commonly outlive their husbands. Women are also more likely to be institutionalized for similar reasons. In the next 40 years, the number of elderly persons in the U.S. is expected to double.

180. The answer is C. *(Wilson, 12/e, pp 1359–1360.)* Gallstones are extremely common; about 20 percent of women and 8 percent of men over the age of 40 have them. Although most gallstones contain cholesterol, elevated levels of plasma cholesterol are not associated with an increased risk. Not only are diabetics at an increased risk of developing gallstones, they also have an increased morbidity and mortality associated with the disease. Chronic hemolytic anemia predisposes to the formation of calcium bilirubinate gallstones, which are more common in Asia. Additional risk factors for gallstones include age, obesity, and chronic biliary infection.

181. The answer is C. *(Wyngaarden, 19/e, p 2012.)* Although systemic lupus erythematosus (SLE) is predominantly a disease of young women, it is much less common than rheumatoid arthritis in this age group. The female:male ratio is about 10:1. The black:white ratio is about 3:1 in the U.S. A black woman in the U.S. has about a 1 in 250 chance of developing lupus in her lifetime. Diagnosis is based on fulfilling at least 4 out of 11 criteria (such as the presence of pleurisy or pericarditis) but does not require a positive ANA test.

182. The answer is B. *(Wilson, 12/e, p 1526.)* Folate deficiency can occur because of insufficient intake in the diet, because of malabsorption, or because of increased needs for the vitamin. Folate is found in green, leafy vegetables; strict vegetarians are at risk of deficiency of cobalamin (vitamin B_{12}), which is found in meats. Persons with chronic hemolysis, such as those with sickle cell anemia, can have increased needs for folate. Dialysis increases the need for the water-soluble (and dialyzable) vitamins.

183. The answer is E. *(Wyngaarden, 19/e, p 576.)* Chronic renal failure is associated with accelerated atherogenesis; dialysis does not appear to slow this process. Overall mortality for patients on dialysis is approximately 5 percent per year. Depression is common. Infections with *Staphylococcus aureus*, mycobacteria, and hepatitis B have an increased incidence.

184. The answer is D. *(Wilson, 12/e, p 147.)* Aging is by far the most important risk factor for developing cataracts. Both types of diabetes are complicated by early cataract formation, possibly owing to the effect of hyperglycemia on the lens proteins. Other causes include trauma, ultraviolet radiation, and several congenital infections, such as rubella.

185. The answer is E. *(Wilson, 12/e, pp 1505–1507.)* There are two types of hemophilia: type A, or factor VIII deficiency; and type B, or factor IX deficiency. Both are sex-linked genetic disorders, which indicates that the faulty genes are carried on the X chromosome. Thus, there is no association with environmental factors or with HLA type (which is carried on chromosome 6).

186. The answer is A. *(Wilson, 12/e, pp 1102, 1577.)* In the past 25 years, age-adjusted mortality has increased for certain forms of cancer, including cancer of the lung and pancreas, probably because of cigarette smoking. The mortality from uterine cancer has declined by about 60 percent in that time, mainly owing to increased acceptance and use of the Pap test. Mortality from stomach cancer has also declined by 60 percent; the reason is unknown.

187. The answer is A. *(Wilson, 12/e, pp 1350–1351.)* Hepatoma accounts for only 1 to 2 percent of cancers in the Western world. But in parts of the world where chronic, lifelong carriage of the hepatitis B surface antigen (HBsAg) is common, such as Africa and Asia, hepatoma accounts for approximately 25 percent of all types of malignancy. In the Western world, the tumor is more commonly seen in persons with cirrhosis. Hepatocellular carcinomas are up to four times more common in men than women.

188. The answer is D. *(Wilson, 12/e, pp 682–683.)* Recent studies have shown that infection with HSV-1 is more common and tends to occur earlier in life than infection with HSV-2. Either type of virus can cause oral or genital lesions, but genital HSV-2 infection is eight to ten times more likely to reactivate than genital HSV-1 infection. Previous infection with one type of HSV does not provide protection against subsequent infection with the other type. Reports of HSV-2 infection are twice as common using seroepidemiologic techniques as they are by clinical history. Both viruses may be excreted by asymptomatic persons.

189. The answer is E. *(Wilson, 12/e, pp 1579–1580.)* A higher-than-normal incidence of breast, colon, retinal, and skin cancers has been demonstrated in relatives of patients with these cancers. There are certain inherited syndromes (such as Gardner syndrome) associated with a markedly increased risk of colon cancer (nearly 100 percent). A woman who has a first-degree relative (mother, sister, daughter) with breast cancer has a threefold increased risk of developing the disease. The gene responsible for retinoblastoma is located on chromosome 13. Laryngeal cancer is related to smoking and alcohol use.

190. The answer is E. *(Last, Maxcy-Rosenau, 13/e, pp 818–819.)* The relationship that exists between marital status and cancer of the cervix may be due to the increased sexual activity that usually accompanies marriage and increased exposure to possible carcinogenic agents. This theory is supported by the fact that prostitutes as well as married women have an increased frequency of cancer of the cervix. Endocrine factors may account for the difference in the risk of breast cancer between single and married women; breast cancer is more common among nulliparous women than among women who have borne children. Risk of ovarian cancer is also higher in nulliparous women.

191. The answer is D. *(Wilson, 12/e, p 1102.)* Probably because rates of cigarette smoking in men are lower than they were 20 to 30 years ago, incidence rates of lung cancer are actually on the decline in men. However, smoking rates in women were increasing, at least until very recently, and thus rates of lung cancer continue to rise in women. Lung cancer has replaced breast cancer as the leading cause of cancer death in women.

192. The answer is E. *(Wilson, 12/e, pp 1580–1581.)* Tobacco-related cancers (mainly lung cancer) cause more than 30 percent of all cancer deaths in the U.S. Smoking cigarettes increases the risk of lung cancer at least tenfold. As more women with a long-term smoking history enter the age with the highest incidence rate for lung cancer, rates of tobacco-related cancer among women are increasing. Pancreatic cancer is at least twice as common in smokers; smoking is a risk factor for cancer of the bladder and kidney. Oral, laryngeal, and esophageal cancers are also increased by cigarette smoke, particularly among heavy alcohol drinkers.

193. The answer is E. *(Wilson, 12/e, pp 2039–2040.)* Although the cause of multiple sclerosis is unknown, its epidemiology has been well studied. Women constitute about 60 percent of the cases. In general, the incidence of the disease increases with distance from the equator; the disease is twice as frequent in the northern as in the southern U.S. Certain HLA types, such as B7 in whites and DW2 in blacks, are more common among patients with the disease. First-degree relatives (siblings, parents) of patients with MS are at increased risk of developing the disease compared with the general population. The incidence of multiple sclerosis is lower in blacks than whites for persons living in the same region.

194. The answer is A. *(Wilson, 12/e, p 556.)* While the majority of patients with pneumococcal pneumonia can be cured with appropriate antibiotic therapy, there are several characteristics associated with poor survival. These include patients at extremes of age (either very young or old), underlying conditions (such as alcoholism), and multilobar disease. Leukopenia, but not leukocytosis, is also associated with decreased survival.

195. The answer is A. *(Last, Maxcy-Rosenau, 13/e, p 812.)* The most common cancers in developing countries, in order of frequency of occurrence, are cancers of the uterine cervix, mouth and pharynx, esophagus, breast, and lung.

196. The answer is B. *(Wilson, 12/e, pp 1633–1634.)* Exposure to ultraviolet light is a cause of skin cancer. Both squamous and basal cell tumors can result from chronic exposure. Although skin cancer (not including melanoma) is by far the most common form of cancer, very few patients with skin cancer (about 1 percent) die of the disease. Sun exposure early in life is also associated with melanoma.

197. The answer is E. *(Wilson, 12/e, pp 1384–1385.)* Of 100 patients who have cancer of the pancreas, only 1 to 2 patients can be expected to survive 5 years after diagnosis. Early diagnosis is difficult. Patients may complain of vague abdominal pain or weakness. Tumors of the body and tail of the pancreas are rarely detected before metastases. About 15 to 20 percent of patients who have tumors of the head of the pancreas are surgical candidates for resection. Radiotherapy and chemotherapy do not prolong life.

198. The answer is A. *(Wilson, 12/e, pp 1629–1631.)* More than 90 percent of men have benign prostatic hypertrophy by age 80. Prostate cancer follows lung and colon cancer as a cause of cancer death in U.S. men over 55 years of age. The reason the U.S. incidence of prostate cancer is higher in blacks than in whites is not known.

199. The answer is E. *(Wilson, 12/e, p 1090.)* Conditions and periods associated with a high risk of thromboembolism include the postoperative period, use of oral contraceptives, congestive heart failure, the postpartum period, chronic pulmonary disease, fractures or other injuries of lower extremities, obesity, deep venous insufficiency in the legs, prolonged bed rest, and carcinoma.

200. The answer is C. *(Wilson, 12/e, p 1437.)* The incidence of rheumatoid arthritis is about three times higher in women than in men. Rheumatoid arthritis is nearly four times more common in first-degree relatives of those with the disease, and there is an association with HLA-DR4. Joint destruction is a hallmark of the disease and progresses in most cases. About 80 percent of patients develop evidence of joint destruction after 10 years.

201. The answer is D. *(Wilson, 12/e, p 1475.)* Osteoarthritis (OA) is almost universal by age 75 and the prevalence is similar by sex. While it afflicts all races, the pattern of joint involvement varies. Heberden's nodes (OA of the distal interphalangeal joints) occur at increased frequency in siblings.

202. The answer is C. *(Wilson, 12/e, pp 1977–2002.)* The major risk factors for stroke are hypertension, diabetes, electrocardiographic evidence of an enlarged heart, hypercholesterolemia, and cigarette smoking. The risk increases when one of the factors is present and is further increased if more than one factor is present. There is no evidence that alcoholism is related to increased risk of stroke; and type A personality, although possibly associated with an increased risk of myocardial infarction, has not been related to an increased risk of stroke.

203. The answer is E. *(Wilson, 13/e, pp 1439–1440.)* The course of rheumatoid arthritis is unpredictable but is worse in patients who have certain characteristics, including advanced age. White women are more likely to have progressively worsening disease than are white men. Certain serologic markers, including high titers of rheumatoid factor and high serum haptoglobin levels, are also associated with poor prognosis. There is no relationship with the initial pattern of arthritis.

204. The answer is D. *(Wilson, 12/e, pp 1790–1792.)* The relative increased risk for deep venous thrombosis and pulmonary embolism is from two- to twelvefold in users of oral contraceptives. There is no association between use of oral contraceptives and breast cancer or osteoporosis. The synthetic estrogen diethylstilbestrol (DES) was identified as a transplacental carcinogen. Some daughters of women given the drug during pregnancy to prevent miscarriage subsequently developed adenocarcinoma of the vagina and cervix. However, DES is not an oral contraceptive.

205. The answer is E. *(Last, Maxcy-Rosenau, 13/e, pp 873, 877. Wilson, 12/e, pp 1742–1743.)* Factors that predispose an adult to diabetes mellitus include increased age, familial inheritance, gestational diabetes, and obesity; the last is considered the most important factor. Most adults who have maturity-onset diabetes are obese. Although the precise mode of inheritance is unknown, the genetic association is clear. Nearly one-third of patients' offspring will develop abnormal glucose tolerance or frank diabetes. There is little evidence that increased dietary sugar is a risk factor for diabetes.

206. The answer is C. *(Wilson, 12/e, pp 1074–1082.)* Contributing etiologic factors in chronic bronchitis include air pollution, occupation, infection, smoking, and genotype. Chronic bronchitis is more prevalent in urban regions where air is often polluted. Workers exposed to dusts and some gases have a higher incidence of the disease. Not only is cigarette smoking the most common single etiologic factor, it also potentiates every other factor. It impairs ciliary motility, inhibits fixation of alveolar macrophages, leads to hypertrophy of the glands, and probably causes polymorphonuclear cells to release proteolytic enzymes.

207. The answer is B. *(Wilson, 12/e, p 1971.)* About 2 to 5 percent of children will have a seizure associated with a febrile illness. Fever, trauma, and infections are the most commonly identified causes of seizures in children. Seizures are more likely with slowly growing malignancies. About half of patients with posttraumatic seizures will spontaneously recover.

208. The answer is B. *(Wilson, 12/e, pp 1753–1756.)* Diabetes is the leading cause of blindness in adults in the U.S. More than half of all nontraumatic amputations occur in diabetic persons with nonhealing limb ulcers or gangrene. Other complications include renal failure, coronary artery disease, and stroke.

209. The answer is B. *(Wilson, 12/e, p 1626.)* Testicular cancer is one of the most common malignancies in men between the ages of 20 and 35, when the incidence of the disease peaks; it is uncommon after the age of 40. It is more common in whites than in blacks. Males with intraabdominal testes are at several-fold increased risk. About 6000 males develop the disease each year in the U.S.

210. The answer is A. *(Wilson, 12/e, pp 1063, 2160–2161.)* Passive, or second-hand, exposure to cigarette smoke may lead to increased levels of carbon monoxide. Children born to parents who smoke cigarettes are more likely to develop respiratory illnesses than children of nonsmoking parents. Other exposed nonsmokers may develop conjunctivitis, headache, nasal congestion, and cough. Exposure to cigarette smoke may exacerbate the symptoms of persons with chronic obstructive pulmonary disease (COPD) and angina pectoris. The incidence of lung cancer appears to be increased in nonsmoking persons married to persons who smoke compared with those married to nonsmokers.

211. The answer is E. *(Wyngaarden, 19/e, pp 1014–1022.)* Prognosis of Hodgkin's disease correlates with the stage of the disease at diagnosis. However, weight loss, fever, and chills are usually regarded as unfavorable prognostic signs and symptoms. Histologic types have been associated with their 5-year survival data: patients with the lymphocyte-predominant type have a better survival than those with the other types. Women have a better prognosis than men; the reason is unknown.

212. The answer is C. *(Wilson, 12/e, p 1626.)* Men with a history of cryptorchid (undescended) testes have a several-fold increased risk of developing testicular cancer; patients with intraabdominal testes are at higher risk than those with high inguinal testes. Both the cryptorchid and contralateral (normally placed) testicle are at increased risk. There are two peak incidences of testicular cancer: one in early childhood and a larger one in men 20 to 35 years of age.

213. The answer is C. *(Wilson, 12/e, p 1269.)* Both ulcerative colitis and Crohn's disease are rare; thus, the odds ratio is a valid estimator of the relative risk. Because nearly 90 percent of Americans are white, disease rates in whites will be approximately those seen in the overall population; with a relative risk of 2.0, rates in blacks will be about half of the overall rates. Prevalence is approximately equal to incidence times the duration of disease; the diseases have a similar duration of about 15 years. With a prevalence of 100 per 100,000, there are about 240,000 persons with ulcerative colitis in the U.S. (total population of about 240 million).

214. The answer is B. *(Last, Maxcy-Rosenau, 13/e, pp 407–409.)* Exposure to benzene may occur in solvents, coal, oil, chemicals, pharmaceutical, paint, adhesive, solvent, and pesticide industries. Commercial grades of other aromatic hydrocarbons, such as toluene and xylene, as well as motor fuel also contain significant amounts of benzene. Inhalation of the vapor is the main route of absorption, and retention is highest in adipose tissue and bone marrow. Benzene is a potent myelotoxic agent associated with a dose-dependent incidence of aplastic anemia. Testicular atrophy and chromosomal aberrations have also been reported. Although benzene is absorbed via the lungs, it is not associated with an increased incidence of lung cancer.

215. The answer is D. *(Wilson, 12/e, pp 1527, 2101, 2185.)* Exposure to organic mercury can cause an intention tremor, or even delirium (use of mercury in the manufacture of felt hats led to the phrase "mad as a hatter"). Lead poisoning in adults causes peripheral neuropathy and ataxia; in children it can cause irreversible defects in the central nervous system. Long-term exposure to nitrous oxide (usually as a result of abuse) has been reported to cause a neuropathy similar to that seen in pernicious anemia. Exposure to arsenic can cause delirium or even coma. Exposure to sulfur dioxide mainly causes irritation of the mucous membranes.

216. The answer is C. *(Wilson, 12/e, pp 1058–1060.)* Mesothelioma, a cancer that develops from the mesothelial cells that cover the pleural and other serous membranes, occurs almost exclusively among persons who have been exposed to air containing large numbers of asbestos particles. Pericardial mesothelioma is not associated with asbestos exposure. Cancers of the bronchus and the larynx are most commonly associated with cigarette smoking. Byssinosis is a pneumoconiosis due to chronic inhalation of textile dusts.

217. The answer is A. *(Last, Maxcy-Rosenau, 13/e, pp 386, 387, 391, 411, 419, 627.)* Ethylene glycol, found in antifreeze, causes an acute tubular necrosis usually seen in attempted overdoses. Chronic exposure to cadmium or lead—both of which are used in welding, soldering, and jewelry-making—causes injury to the proximal tubules and may lead to chronic renal failure; acute overexposure has been associated with oliguric renal failure. Halogenated hydrocarbons, such as carbon tetrachloride, cause acute tubular necrosis, especially if exposure is via inhalation. Chlorine reaction products from water disinfection processes are associated with bladder cancer.

218. The answer is E. *(Last, Maxcy-Rosenau, 13/e, p 816. Wilson, 12/e, p 1633.)* More workers are exposed to sunlight than to any of the other carcinogens listed in the question. In occupations related to agriculture, construction, fishing, forestry, gardening, landscaping, and installation of telephone and electric lines, large numbers of workers are exposed to ultraviolet light. Arsenic is the most common chemical carcinogen in skin cancers. Chronic exposure to coal tar and soot can also cause skin cancer.

219. The answer is D. *(Wilson, 12/e, pp 1056–1060.)* Pneumoconiosis, a fibrosing disease of the lungs, usually occurs as a result of occupational exposure to air that contains particulate matter. Anthracosis, silicosis, asbestosis, berylliosis, farmer's lung, and byssinosis are among the more than 30 forms of pneumoconioses that have been described in the literature. Sulfur oxides, nitrogen oxides, oil fumes, and cigarette smoke are likely to cause acute bronchospasm or to exacerbate preexisting diseases such as chronic bronchitis and emphysema.

220. The answer is A. *(Last, Maxcy-Rosenau, 13/e, pp 344–345, 356. Rosenstock, p 42.)* Mesotheliomas of the pleural and peritoneal surfaces are the classic asbestos-related tumors because they are rarely seen in persons never exposed to asbestos. It is important to realize that in persons with asbestosis, however, the principal cause of death is bronchogenic carcinoma. Carcinomas of the colon and larynx are also associated with asbestos exposure. Workers who are exposed to asbestos but who do not smoke have a fivefold increased risk of bronchogenic carcinoma (over nonexposed persons), and workers who are exposed to asbestos and who do smoke have a fifty- to one-hundred-fold increased risk.

221. The answer is C. (*Last, Maxcy-Rosenau, 13/e, pp 414–415.*) Neither polyvinyl chloride (PVC) nor the vinyl chloride monomer from which it is derived has been clearly shown to cause lung disease. Exposure to PVC causes a bone syndrome with resorption and spontaneous fractures of the distal phalanges (called *acroosteolysis*). PVC can cause hemangiosarcomas and nonmalignant liver disease with associated portal hypertension.

222. The answer is C. (*Last, Maxcy-Rosenau, 13/e, pp 513–522.*) Nonionizing radiation does not cause molecular ionization or disruption of atomic nuclei. It includes extremely low-frequency electromagnetic fields, radiowaves, microwaves, and infrared, visible, and ultraviolet radiation. Epidemiological studies of extremely low-frequency radiation (electromagnetic fields) suggest exposure may be associated with leukemia, lymphoma, and tumors of the nervous system. They also suggest that exposure to electromagnetic fields from video display terminals during pregnancy may cause miscarriages and birth defects, but not sterility.

223. The answer is C. (*Last, Maxcy-Rosenau, 13/e, pp 551–552.*) Mining and quarrying is the most dangerous industry in the United States. Agriculture is second; about 50 deaths per 100,000 workers occur each year. According to recent estimates, about 109 million disabling injuries and 11,000 deaths occur annually in industrial occupations.

224. The answer is D. (*Last, Maxcy-Rosenau, 13/e, p 918.*) A strong correlation exists between the level of serum uric acid and both the prevalence and incidence of gout. Serum uric acid is elevated in males and by use of alcohol and diuretics. Exposure to lead is also associated with gout.

225. The answer is B. (*Last, Maxcy-Rosenau, 13/e, pp 1023–1027.*) Over 2.8 million people were hospitalized for injuries each year from

1983 to 1987. Injury-related direct medical costs amounted to almost $45 billion in 1985. Motor vehicles account for over 50 percent of injury-related deaths in the U.S.

226. The answer is D. *(Wilson, 12/e, p 1058.)* A common finding in people who have been exposed chronically to asbestos is calcification of the pleura and diaphragm. The pleural calcification is often unilateral. The pattern of calcification is unique and easily differentiated from that caused by trauma and surgery. Calcification of the diaphragm is so rare that this finding is almost pathognomonic for asbestosis. Bilateral fibrosis is not a specific finding in the diagnosis of asbestosis. Although pleural effusion is not specific, its presence in a patient with asbestosis should prompt a search for bronchogenic carcinoma or mesothelioma.

227. The answer is C. *(Last, Maxcy-Rosenau, 13/e, pp 100–102. Neinstein, 5/e, pp 725–726.)* Although the absolute numbers of most STDs are highest in those 20 to 24 years old, adolescents 15 to 19 years of age have the highest rates of STDs when these rates are corrected to include only sexually active persons. Low-income, minority heterosexuals have the highest rates of STDs in the U.S. Cervicitis is usually asymptomatic. Adolescents frequently have cervical ectopy; *N. gonorrhoeae* and *C. trachomatis* have a predilection for columnar epithelium such as that present in cervical ectopy.

228. The answer is B. *(Last, Maxcy-Rosenau, 13/e, pp 365–370. Wilson, 12/e, p 1059.)* This condition was noted to occur even in coal workers exposed to dust virtually free of silica. Anthracite dust is more dangerous for two reasons: (1) the smaller particle size causes more extensive scar formation; and (2) anthracite deposits are associated with higher levels of silica dust. Progressive massive fibrosis occurs in only a minority of cases. Coal workers pneumoconiosis, or "black lung," develops in 12 percent of all miners and up to 50 percent of anthracite miners with more than 20 years of dust exposure.

229. The answer is C. *(Wilson, 12/e, p 2185.)* Differences in the biologic properties of inorganic and organic compounds of mercury have been learned through pollution studies, such as the study of the accidental poisonings that occurred in Minamata Bay, Japan. Methyl mercury collects in nervous system tissue and results in mild to severe neurological disorders from atrophy of cells of the cerebellum and cerebral cortex. It also passes through the placenta and breast milk; children and fetuses are especially susceptible to its neurological effects. Gingivitis may be caused by inorganic, but not organic compounds.

230. The answer is D. *(Wilson, 12/e, pp 1739–1759.)* In the U.S. the leading cause of ESRD is diabetes, followed by hypertension, glomerulonephritis, cystic kidney disease, and other urologic diseases. In 1988 over 175,000 patients received treatment for ESRD, 8932 renal transplants were performed, and over 35,000 patients had functioning renal transplants.

231. The answer is C. *(Last, Maxcy-Rosenau, 13/e, p 389.)* It is important to distinguish between exposures to organic and inorganic lead because they cause different syndromes. Acute overexposure to inorganic lead causes predominantly gastrointestinal symptoms. Chronic exposure causes anemia and encephalopathy. Overexposure to organic lead causes a syndrome limited to the central nervous system, with insomnia, anorexia, irritability, and eventually an agitated encephalopathy. It is usually seen in workers who have been cleaning gasoline storage tanks. Gasoline station attendants are exposed to an organic lead compound, tetraethyl lead, used as an antiknock ingredient in gasoline, although they rarely develop symptoms of toxicity from this exposure.

232. The answer is D. *(Wilson, 12/e, p 1550.)* The gene frequency for beta thalassemia approaches 0.1 percent in southern Italy and certain Mediterranean islands; it is also prevalent in central Africa, Asia, the South Pacific, and certain parts of India. It is rare in persons of Middle Eastern heritage.

233. The answer is E. *(Last, Maxcy-Rosenau, 13/e, p 523.)* A sudden loud noise can cause a punctured eardrum, which may result in a hearing loss of 20 or more decibels if the puncture is large enough. Continuous noise can cause about twice the amount of hearing loss as intermittent sound, since intermittent sound allows the hearing functions some opportunity to recover. The greatest loss of hearing occurs in the first hour of exposure and then levels off. The spectrum of the noise is also important: at the same intensity, low-frequency sounds are less damaging than high-frequency sounds. The intensity and duration of sound are the primary determinants of hearing impairment. For noises of the same intensity, impulsive sounds such as gunshots generally pose a greater risk than continuous noise. The tonality of sounds does not affect hearing.

234. The answer is C. *(Wilson, 12/e, p 1408.)* Persistent diarrhea is frequent in AIDS patients, and *Cryptosporidium, Isospora belli, Salmonella,* and cytomegaloviruses are the common etiologic agents. *Toxoplasmosis gondii* is one of the most common central nervous system infections in persons with AIDS.

235. The answer is C. *(Wilson, 12/e, pp 651–661.)* Congenital syphilis is acquired from transplacental or perinatal transmission of *Treponema pallidum.* Tetracycline is not recommended in pregnancy because of potential adverse effects to the fetus; erythromycin should be used only in patients who have documented penicillin allergy and who are not candidates for desensitization. All women should be screened serologically for syphilis early in pregnancy with a nontreponemal test (VDRL or RPR); high-risk women should be screened again at 28 weeks and delivery.

236. The answer is E. *(Wilson, 12/e, pp 707–708.)* Serologic studies indicate that 10 to 20 percent of young adults are susceptible to rubella in the U.S. Congenital rubella syndrome occurs in 25 percent or more of infants born to women who develop rubella during the first trimester of pregnancy. Ophthalmological, cardiac, auditory, and neurological anomalies are common. Hutchinson's teeth are anomalous teeth found with congenital syphilis.

237. The answer is D. *(Last, Maxcy-Rosenau, 13/e, pp 371–379.)* Silicosis is a nonimmunological fibrotic lung disease that develops when crystalline silicon dioxide is inhaled. Silicosis is usually characterized by the development of pulmonary nodules, which may coalesce and cause progressive massive fibrosis. Pathologic changes in lung tissue may precede radiographic findings by several years; thus a normal chest radiograph does not exclude the existence of silicosis in a person with significant exposure. Patients have generally been exposed to silica dusts for many years. However, an intense exposure can cause an acute and fulminant form of silicosis, which can be fatal. Occupations that entail risk include mining, sand-blasting (sand is largely composed of quartz), construction, and ceramics.

238. The answer is C. *(Kaplan, 5/e, pp 1821–1837.)* Behavioral problems, including attention-deficit disorders and learning disabilities, are the most prevalent mental health disorders in children; they occur in approximately 10 percent of children. Approximately 0.05 percent of children suffer from autism and 1 percent from mental retardation. Schizophrenia classically occurs later in life.

239. The answer is C. *(Last, Maxcy-Rosenau, 13/e, p 851. Wilson, 12/e, p 189.)* Although dementia is present in 30 to 40 percent of patients with AIDS infections, Alzheimer's disease accounts for 50 to 90 percent of dementia in the western world. Alzheimer's disease is more common among relatives of patients with the disease.

240. The answer is D. *(Kaplan, 5/e, pp 1086–1096.)* It is unknown whether the prevalence of homosexuality in the U.S. is increasing. Most observers believe that the prevalence is constant, but that increasing openness and acceptance have given the appearance of an increased prevalence. Surveys estimate that about 2 percent of women and 4 to 6 percent of men in the U.S. are homosexual.

241. The answer is B. *(Kaplan, 5/e, pp 642–664.)* About 50 percent of the men and 70 percent of the women undergoing treatment for opiate addiction suffer from a major depressive disorder. Other common psychiatric disorders include alcoholism and antisocial personalities. Schizophrenia and mania are rare (less than 1 percent).

242. The answer is C. *(Kaplan, 5/e, pp 1414–1427.)* Completed suicide rates are higher in white males than in white females or in nonwhites of both sexes. The suicide rate increases markedly among elderly white males but not in females or in nonwhites. Males make fewer suicide attempts than females. Suicide rates correlate not only with age, sex, and race but also with marital status (the suicide rate is higher in single, separated, divorced, or widowed persons than in those who are still married), socioeconomic status (especially among poor, elderly white males), psychiatric history, and place of residence.

243. The answer is A. *(Wilson, 12/e, pp 2184–2185.)* Ingestion of paint chips containing lead or of soil and household dust contaminated with lead is a substantial problem in children living in or around buildings that were erected (and painted) more than 30 years ago, when the use of lead-based paints was common. Diagnosis is easy: there are very high levels of free erythrocyte protoporphyrin (FEP) and elevated blood levels of lead. The effects on the developing central nervous system are irreversible. Lead crosses the placenta and may be found in breast milk.

244. The answer is C. *(Kaplan, 5/e, pp 308–326.)* The President's Commission on Mental Health estimated in 1978 that 20 to 30 million Americans needed some form of help for mental and emotional disorders. Studies of patients using medical facilities indicate that 1 out of every 10 had a mental or emotional disorder.

245. The answer is A. *(Kaplan, 5/e, pp 699–705.)* Schizophrenia has a high incidence among persons in their early twenties, while affective psychosis afflicts persons in their late twenties. The annual incidence rate for schizophrenia is approximately 1 per 1000 persons in the 15 to 24 age group. Involutional melancholia and agitated depression are specific types of depression and have their highest incidence in older persons.

246. The answer is B. *(Wilson, 12/e, p 2146.)* Significant impairment of motor coordination can occur with blood alcohol levels of only 20 to 30 mg/dL. However, the legal limit in most states is 100 mg/dL (0.1 percent). Levels of more than 300 to 400 mg/dL can be lethal. Ethanol either alone or with other intoxicants causes more toxic overdose deaths than any other agent.

247. The answer is E. *(Behrman, 14/e, pp 1292–1294.)* While lymphoma is the most prevalent cancer, leukemia is the number one cause of cancer death in adolescents, followed by CNS tumors, bone and joint tumors, lymphomas, and ovarian and testicular neoplasms. The top three causes of death for those aged 15 to 24 are unintentional injuries, homicide, and suicide.

248. The answer is E. *(Kaplan, 5/e, pp 686–698.)* There are 5 to 9 million alcoholics in the U.S. The incidence of alcoholism is higher among men than women; high school dropouts have the highest rate among educational subgroups. Persons with certain occupations, such as bartenders and musicians, are also at higher risk of being alcoholic. About half of the alcohol consumed in this country is drunk by 10 percent of the population.

249. The answer is E. *(Kaplan, 5/e, pp 686–698.)* Alcoholism is four times more common in families with a history of problem drinking, even if the child was adopted out of the family. About half of all alcoholics have such a family history. There is also a markedly increased risk in twins of alcoholics, especially monozygotic twins. The usual age of onset of alcoholism is between 20 and 30; it is rare for the age of onset to be after 65.

250. The answer is D. *(Kaplan, 5/e, pp 1772–1787.)* Although in several early studies, the parents of autistic children were identified frequently as professional people or as having cold or obsessive natures, or both, these findings have not been substantiated in recent studies. In fact, autistic children come from all types of backgrounds, emotional settings, and socioeconomic levels; and autism now is thought to be caused by organic biologic-neurologic factors. Three to four times as many males suffer from the disorder as females.

251. The answer is A. *(Kaplan, 5/e, pp 1414–1427.)* The incidence of suicide increases with age, especially in whites. The highest suicide rate is found in white males of the geriatric population. Married persons are less likely to commit suicide than single persons.

252. The answer is C. *(Kaplan, 5/e, pp 1414–1427.)* The incidence of suicide increases with increasing age; and the rate ranges from less than 1 per 100,000 persons in the group 5 to 14 years of age to greater than 40 per 100,000 persons over 75 years of age. Suicide "attempts," however, occur mainly in young people, and the peak incidence occurs in persons who are in their late teens and early twenties. In the group 6 to 17 years of age, 25 percent of self-poisonings are said to be suicide attempts.

253. The answer is E. *(Last, Maxcy-Rosenau, 13/e, pp 1054–1056.)* The highest risk of suicide in the U.S. is found among persons who are not religious, or who practice Buddhism. Catholics and Jews, especially if they are practicing, are at the lowest risk. Protestants are at intermediate risk.

254. The answer is E. *(Wilson, 12/e, pp 466, 1545.)* Sickle cell patients develop functional asplenia from recurrent splenic infarction. This results in an impaired immune response to polysaccharide antigens such as those of *Streptococcus pneumoniae, Haemophilus influenzae,* and *Neisseria meningitidis.* Persons with functional splenectomy are also at increased risk for fulminant infection with *Babesia microti* and *Plasmodium malariae.*

255. The answer is E. *(Last, Maxcy-Rosenau, 13/e, pp 688–695.)* Although there is an extensive literature on social determinants of disease, very little is known about how such factors work. Virtually all studies have found that four factors—female sex, being married, higher socioeconomic status, and a greater number of social ties—are associated with reduced mortality from nearly all diseases. These relationships are not altered by traditional risk factors (such as blood pressure) or by race or access to care.

256. The answer is C. *(Kaplan, 5/e, pp 664–668.)* The group of people who most commonly have problems of chronic barbiturate abuse are middle-aged, middle-class persons. Heroin addicts use barbiturates as a substitute for, or an enhancer of, heroin. The most common pattern of barbiturate abuse among teenagers is episodic use.

257. The answer is A. *(Kaplan, 5/e, pp 2014–2034.)* Involutional depression appears during the later years of life. The peak incidence for schizophrenia occurs in persons aged 15 to 24 years. Anxiety and obsessive-compulsive disorders usually begin in adolescence or young adulthood.

258. The answer is A. *(Kaplan, 5/e, pp 1096–1103.)* Men who abuse their spouses are rarely prosecuted. Abuse of women in childhood is not associated with a greater probability of being assaulted by a spouse; however, women whose mothers suffered physical abuse are more likely to experience such assault. Wife beating occurs in families of all races, religions, and socioeconomic backgrounds.

259. The answer is B. *(Kaplan, 5/e, pp 1854–1864.)* Anorexia nervosa is characterized by altered perception of body image leading to severe weight loss. About 95 percent of the cases occur in females. Despite the name, anorexia (loss of appetite) is rare initially. Most cases begin between ages 13 and 16.

260. The answer is A. *(Kaplan, 5/e, pp 299–307.)* The prevalence of alcoholism and drug abuse has been shown to be five times greater among males than females. While affective disorders afflict females at a rate about twice that for males, schizophrenia occurs in males and females at about the same rate.

261. The answer is C. *(Wilson, 12/e, p 2131.)* Panic disorders are as common in men as in women. They are estimated to occur in 1 to 2 percent of the population. Their usual age of onset is in the late teens or early twenties. There is a definite familial aggregation of the disorder;

Preventive Medicine and Public Health

up to 18 percent of patients' first-degree relatives will also have panic disorder.

262. The answer is D. *(Kaplan, 5/e, pp 852–858.)* Studies of emotional disturbances in the postpartum period have no relationship with sex of the child, parity, and a variety of other factors. Their cause is unknown but is probably related to hormonal changes. Postpartum depression, the most common manifestation, may last up to 4 weeks. Between 20 and 40 percent of mothers report emotional or cognitive problems post partum.

263. The answer is D. *(Kaplan, 5/e, pp 1962–1970.)* Child abuse is a major problem in the U.S.—up to a million children are maltreated each year, which results in from 2000 to 4000 deaths. Child abusers come from all social classes and educational backgrounds. The mother is more commonly the abuser, perhaps because of greater contact with the child. Abusing parents are usually psychologically immature and have poor impulse control.

264. The answer is B. *(Kaplan, 5/e, pp 642–664.)* Three to four percent of young adults (ages 18 to 25) in the U.S. have had some experience with heroin. The male to female ratio, at least in urban settings, is about 3 to 1. Use of opioids other than heroin is also more common among males. Nearly 5 percent of enlisted personnel in the military reported some use of opioids in the previous 12 months.

265. The answer is B. *(Kaplan, 5/e, pp 1810–1812.)* The cause of stuttering is not known, but genetic factors are thought to be important. Stuttering is two to three times more common in males than females and is also more common among nonwhites. The incidence is highest in young children, although there is a secondary rise in middle-age. There is a strong family tendency to stutter: up to half of the relatives of stutterers have speech dysfluency.

266. The answer is D. *(Kaplan, 5/e, pp 1414–1427.)* Attempted (unsuccessful) suicide is about 10 to 20 times more common than completed suicide. Only 1 to 2 percent of persons who attempt suicide, however, go on to commit suicide. Attempted suicide is more commonly seen in persons with hysterical or antisocial personalities.

267. The answer is D. *(Last, Maxcy-Rosenau, 13/e, pp 948–950.)* A similar proportion (about one in five) of men and women surveyed were affected by a significant mental disorder within the previous 6 months, but the leading diagnoses differed by sex. Phobias were the leading problem in women of all ages, affecting about 10 percent. Problems with alcohol abuse were the most common problem in men ages 18 to 64 (affecting about 10 percent). However, over the age of 65, cognitive impairment was the leading problem: it affected almost 6 percent of men, whereas only 3 percent of men over 65 admitted problems with alcohol. The majority of persons whose responses indicated one or more mental health disorders were not receiving any mental health care.

268. The answer is C. *(Wilson, 12/e, pp 1211–1212.)* Occupational exposures (especially to aromatic amines, aniline dyes, and related organic nitrogen compounds) and cigarette smoking are major risk factors for bladder cancer. There is usually a long latent period, from 15 to 40 years, between exposure and disease. Workers in the rubber industry are exposed to β-naphthylamine, an antioxidant and known carcinogen. Squamous cell carcinoma occurs more frequently in persons with chronic schistosomal infection than in the general population.

269. The answer is B. *(Wilson, 12/e, pp 1608–1612.)* Hodgkin's disease is more prevalent in males. The age-specific incidence curve is bimodal, with an initial peak in persons 15 to 35 years of age and a second peak after age 50. There is an increased risk of Hodgkin's disease in patients with immunodeficiencies and autoimmune diseases. Infection with the Epstein-Barr virus is associated with Burkitt's lymphoma, a non-Hodgkin's lymphoma.

270. The answer is B. *(Wilson, 12/e, pp 1921–1926.)* Most cases of osteoporosis are idiopathic. Factors associated with development of osteoporosis include female gender, postmenopausal state, white race, alcoholism, and low calcium intake during adolescence.

271. The answer is E. *(Last, Maxcy-Rosenau, 13/e, pp 574–576.)* Shift work, night work, work that extends beyond 8 h per day or 40 h per week, heavy lifting, and prolonged standing have all been associated with preterm labor. Studies have found, however, that third-trimester employment in and of itself does not shorten the length of gestation.

272. The answer is D. *(Wilson, 12/e, pp 637–645.)* The time from infection to the development of a positive skin test is between 2 and 8 weeks. The immunosuppression of HIV infection can lead to reactivation of latent tuberculosis; tuberculosis is often the AIDS-defining illness in these patients.

273.   The answer is C. *(Last, Maxcy-Rosenau, 13/e, pp 550–551.)* Over 1 million adolescent women aged 15 to 19 years became pregnant in the U.S. in 1987. Approximately 25 percent of teen births are from repeat pregnancies. The pregnancy rate of U.S. teens is two to three times that of adolescents in Britain, France, Canada, and Sweden.

274–277.   The answers are 274-B, 275-C, 276-A, 277-D. *(Benenson, 15/e, pp 115–117, 182–185, 197–200, 247–250. Last, Maxcy-Rosenau, 13/e, pp 207–210.)* Hepatitis A virus spreads readily in day-care centers, particularly those caring for toddlers in diapers. It usually causes mild or no disease in the children, but may cause significant morbidity in adult contacts.

Cytomegalovirus (CMV) is very common in children in day-care centers; in one study more than half of the children excreted CMV over the course of a year, compared with less than 10 percent of children cared for at home. Most infections are asymptomatic, but infection of the fetus can cause microcephaly, mental retardation, deafness, and death.

Giardiasis affects both children and their adult contacts. Symptoms may be absent, mild, or severe and may include diarrhea, bloating, fat malabsorption, and weight loss. Diagnosis is by identification of cysts or trophozoites in the stool (but false negatives are frequent), or by finding trophozoites in duodenal fluid, either by direct aspiration or with a string test.

Leptospirosis is a systemic illness caused by the spirochete *Leptospira interrogans* and is acquired by contact of abraded skin or mucous membranes with fresh water contaminated with the urine of infected animals. Transmission from person to person is rare. Doxycycline is effective treatment when given early in the course.

278–280.   The answers are 278-D, 279-B, 280-C. *(Mausner, 2/e, pp 78–79, 85–87.)* Meningococcal meningitis, because of its severity and the fear of epidemics, is reportable in all states. Reporting of meningococcal meningitis to local and state health departments by physicians tends to be more complete than reporting of less severe diseases such as measles, German measles, or salmonellosis. Many states improve the completeness of their infectious disease surveillance by requiring all diagnostic laboratories to report the isolation of certain pathogenic microbes.

The incidence and prevalence of chronic diseases such as arthritis are difficult to determine because patients who have arthritis often do not need hospitalization. The National Health Interview Survey uses data obtained by conducting household surveys of defined populations and attempts continuously to provide data on the health status and needs of the country.

In several states and foreign countries, all newly diagnosed cases of cancer that occur in a defined geographic area are reported to a cancer registry and then followed by the registry until death of the patients. Such registries provide very important information on the incidence, prevalence, and survival rates of different types of cancers. In addition, the registries provide a source of cases for case-control studies and other research.

281–284. The answers are 281-B, 282-D, 283-A, 284-C. *(Benenson, 15/e, pp 66, 83, 224, 271, 330, 347–348, 353–354, 381–382, 386, 392, 411–417, 486.)* Rabies, psittacosis, and salmonellosis are zoonoses, that is, infections transmitted from animals to humans. The reservoirs of rabies include domestic and wild canines, cats, skunks, raccoons, bats, and other biting mammals. Psittacosis is a zoonosis involving birds such as parakeets, parrots, pigeons, turkeys, and other domestic fowl. *Salmonella* species infect poultry, rodents, dogs, cats, and birds (*S. typhi* is an exception in that no animal hosts are known).

Influenza, yellow fever, and chickenpox are caused by viruses. The diseases differ significantly in their clinical manifestations: influenza is an acute respiratory tract infection; chickenpox is characterized by fever and a typical skin rash; and yellow fever is a severe disseminated viral infection with jaundice.

Pneumococcus, Streptococcus, and *Brucella* are genera of bacteria. Microbes of the first two genera are pathogens responsible for respiratory tract infections in humans. *Brucella* is a cause of widespread zoonoses in cattle, pigs, goats, and sheep, but only occasionally causes human disease.

Measles, shigellosis, and scabies can be transmitted directly from person to person. Measles virus is spread in the respiratory secretions of infected persons; shigellosis is easily caused by ingestion of only a few hundred *Shigella* bacteria and can be spread from person to person by the fecal-oral route; and scabies, a skin infection caused by the mite *Sarcoptes scabiei,* is spread by direct person-to-person contact, often during sexual activity.

285–288. The answers are 285-A, 286-B, 287-D, 288-C. *(Mausner, 2/e, pp 268–269.)* *Immunogenicity* is a term that describes the ability of a microbe or purified antigen to induce specific antibody production in a host as a result of infection or immunization. For example, measles virus is very immunogenic because most persons develop neutralizing antibody, which persists for life following a single infection.

Pathogenicity is the capacity of a microbe to cause symptomatic illness in an infected host. The enormous numbers of nonpathogenic bacteria (up to 10^{10} per gram of colonic contents) present in the human body and the normal flora on the human body's external surface do not cause disease.

Virulence refers to the severity of illness produced by a microbe and is measured by the percentage of severe or fatal cases. Virulence may vary depending on the defenses of the host; for example, malnutrition impairs defenses against infection. In malnourished children, measles has a case-fatality rate of up to 10 percent compared with less than 0.1 percent in well-nourished children.

Contagiousness of a microbe refers to the ability of a microbe to spread in a population of exposed susceptible persons. The secondary attack rate, that is, the incidence of a disease in contacts of a case, often is used to assess contagiousness.

289–292. The answers are 289-A, 290-C, 291-B, 292-D. *(Benenson, 15/e, pp 61–66, 130–132, 170–175.)* Staphylococcal food poisoning is caused by a heat-stable enterotoxin produced when staphylococci multiply in food. The incubation period is usually 2 to 4 h, and the illness is characterized by the sudden onset of severe nausea, vomiting, cramps, prostration, and diarrhea.

Botulism is caused by a toxin produced by *Clostridium botulinum*. The toxin, produced anaerobically in improperly processed foods, is neurotoxic, and the illness is characterized by progressive descending muscle paralysis. Botulism may lead to death from respiratory failure.

Food poisoning caused by *Clostridium perfringens* usually has an incubation period of 10 to 12 h and is characterized by abrupt onset of abdominal colic followed by diarrhea. Vomiting is unusual, and the disease is usually of short duration. Outbreaks result from contamination of food during preparation and by improper cooking and storage; these circumstances allow bacteria to multiply.

Most cases of traveler's diarrhea are caused by enterotoxin-producing strains of *Escherichia coli*. Although the mechanism of action of *E. coli* enterotoxin is similar to that of cholera enterotoxin, disease due to the former is usually not as severe. Disease due to *E. coli* enterotoxin is most common in regions of the world where adequate sanitation and pure water supplies are absent.

293–296. The answers are 293-A, 294-E, 295-C, 296-B. *(Wilson, 12/e, pp 1437, 1463–1464, 1475, 1834–1835.)* Gout is caused by the deposition of urate crystals in a joint. It is always associated with hyperuricemia, which is frequently caused by diuretic therapy used in the treatment of hypertension or congestive heart failure. It can also be idiopathic (caused by either overproduction or underexcretion of uric acid) or associated with underlying malignancy or renal disease.

The onset of rheumatoid arthritis is most frequent during the fourth and fifth decades of life and is associated with HLA-DR4.

Osteoarthritis afflicts the majority of persons over the age of 75 years and is by far the most common form of arthritis in all regions of the U.S.

Although sarcoidosis may be slightly more common in the southeastern U.S. than in other regions, it is still a rare disease.

297–300. The answers are 297-E, 298-B, 299-E, 300-B. *(Wilson, 12/e, pp 692, 1351, 1457.)* The hepatitis B virus, a mostly double-stranded DNA virus, has been associated with both hepatomas and polyarteritis nodosa (PAN). Hepatomas are most commonly seen among persons who are chronic carriers of hepatitis B. PAN is a systemic vasculitis of small and medium-sized arteries and is manifested by involvement of multiple organ systems. The nature of the relationship between the hepatitis B virus and PAN is not clear; however, approximately 30 percent of patients with PAN are HBsAg-positive.

Epstein-Barr virus, a member of the herpes family, is the cause of infectious mononucleosis. High titers of antibody to certain of the viral antigens are seen in the majority of patients with anaplastic nasopharyngeal cancer (a relatively common cancer in southeast China) and with Burkitt's lymphoma. Interestingly, there does not seem to be as strong a relationship between Burkitt's lymphoma and EBV in the U.S. Varicella-zoster virus and hepatitis A and E viruses are generally not associated with chronic disease.

301–305. The answers are 301-B, 302-A, 303-E, 304-D, 305-C. *(Last, Maxcy-Rosenau, 13/e, pp 367–466. Wilson, 12/e, pp 1053–1063.)* Occupational exposure to beryllium dust is a hazard to workers who manufacture aircraft, radar equipment, and fluorescent lamps and in some metallurgical processes. Noncaseating granulomas are the consequence of long exposure to beryllium dust. These are followed by a diffuse interstitial fibrosis that reduces lung volume, decreases gas transport, and causes dyspnea and nonproductive cough.

The acute symptoms of byssinosis occur in many workers after years of breathing air that contains dusts of cotton, flax, or hemp and consist of episodic obstruction with chest tightness, cough, and wheezing. In persons who have chronic byssinosis, the pulmonary damage is irreversible.

Rheumatoid pneumoconiosis, or Caplan's syndrome, is seen occasionally in coal workers. Pulmonary nodules are accompanied by seropositive rheumatoid arthritis. This syndrome may also occur with silicosis and other pneumoconioses.

Siderosis is caused by chronic inhalation of iron oxide dust that is airborne in the work environment of welders. Pulmonary function and tissue responses are generally not significant, but striking changes may be seen on chest radiograph.

Hypersensitivity pneumonia is an immunologically induced alveolitis secondary to repeated inhalations of organic dusts. "Farmer's lung" occurs with inhalation of actinomycetes, which may be found in hay, grain, and silage.

306–310. The answers are 306-A, 307-E, 308-D, 309-B, 310-C. *(Wilson, 12/e, pp 625–626, 635, 745, 749, 1326–1327.)* Although most occupational diseases are not infectious in origin, it is important to be aware of those that are. Butchers, meat packers, farmers, and livestock handlers are at risk of developing brucellosis, a febrile illness caused by several species of *Brucella,* a gram-negative coccobacillus. Occupational infection usually results from inoculation through abraded skin or mucous membranes; gloves and goggles can prevent this form of spread. Infection may also result from ingestion of raw milk or animal tissues. Treatment is with tetracycline.

Sporotrichosis is caused by the fungus *Sporothrix schenckii,* a common plant saprophyte. Infection is usually caused by inoculation of the organism into a wound, such as that caused by a rose thorn. It usually causes a lymphangitic disease, with a localized papule and distant nodules. Treatment is with oral potassium iodide.

Air-conditioning workers and others (such as hospital patients) exposed to air from cooling ducts containing water are susceptible to legionellosis, a severe pneumonia caused by *Legionella pneumophila. L. pneumophila* is a gram-negative rod that inhabits warm, moist areas, such as cooling systems. It is named after a famous epidemic that occurred in 1976 at an American Legion convention in Philadelphia, in which at least 220 people were infected with a (then) mysterious illness. Treatment is with erythromycin.

Dentists and other health workers exposed to blood and other body fluids are at risk for hepatitis B, a viral infection. The incubation period is 1 to 4 months. There is no treatment, but the disease can be prevented by immunization.

Spelunkers are at risk for histoplasmosis, a fungal infection caused by *Histoplasma capsulatum*. *H. capsulatum* grows in soil, particularly that enriched by bird or bat excrement (the reason it is found in caves). Infection, which is more common in the central and southeastern U.S., is usually asymptomatic but may cause a chronic pulmonary disease that mimics tuberculosis. Treatment is with ketoconazole or amphotericin B.

311–315. The answers are 311-E, 312-A, 313-A, 314-D, 315-B. *(Last, Maxcy-Rosenau, 13/e, pp 359, 372, 463.)* The principal health hazard associated with pottery and glass manufacture is silicosis (nodular pulmonary fibrosis) due to inhalation of silica dust generated during the manufacturing process. Hydrogen sulfide, methane, and carbon dioxide asphyxiant gases are generated from manure or sewage and pose occupational hazards if ventilation is poor. Welding burns organic material with oxygen to produce carbon monoxide, and if ventilation is restricted asphyxiation will occur. The Environmental Protection Agency's ban on asbestos provided for a 7-year phase-out period; brake blocks, pipes, and shingles will not be affected until 1996.

316–319. The answers are 316-E, 317-E, 318-B, 319-A. *(Last, Maxcy-Rosenau, 13/e, pp 46–48.)* Deaths associated with automobile crashes account for about 20 percent of all deaths in children 1 to 14 years old. In this age group, injuries of all types caused almost 50 percent of all deaths. Cancer is the second leading cause of death. One-third of the deaths in the age group 14 to 24 are due to automobile crashes. Cancer is also the second leading cause of death in this age group. The leading cause of death in the group 25 to 44 years of age is cancer, only slightly ahead of heart disease. Heart disease is the leading cause of death for adults in the group 45 to 64 years of age. For these adults, cancer is the second leading cause of death and the death rate for stroke exceeds that for automobile crashes. The only infectious disease listed among the ten leading causes of death is pneumonia, which outranks automobile crashes as a cause of death only in infants less than 1 year of age and in adults over 65 years of age.

320–324. The answers are 320-C, 321-E, 322-D, 323-D, 324-D. *(Last, Maxcy-Rosenau, 13/e, pp 422, 816.)* Of the over 70,000 chemicals currently in commercial production, approximately 2 percent have been tested for their carcinogenicity. Of these, about 50 have been found by direct observations of exposed human populations to cause cancer. β-*Naphthylamine,* an aromatic amine used to produce dyes, rubber, and many other chemicals, has been identified as an agent that causes bladder cancer. *Benzene,* or benzol, is used in coal and oil derivatives, solvents, pesticides, and pharmaceuticals. Based on epidemiological evidence, benzene is a causative agent of leukemia. Vapors of *nickel,* a component of many alloys, and nickel sulfides, when inhaled over long periods of time, have been cited as a cause of cancer of the nasal cavities and the lungs. Workers in the *chromate*-producing industries such as the steel industry are at high risk of developing cancer of the nasal cavities and lungs. Asbestos exposure is associated with excess cases of lung cancer and mesothelioma.

325–328. The answers are 325-C, 326-A, 327-A, 328-C. *(Last, 13/e, pp 741–742. Wilson, 12/e, pp 1233, 1248, 1922, 2160.)* Alcohol and tobacco both cause esophageal cancer. The risk of the disease is increased in smokers about fivefold and in drinkers about tenfold. Persons who both smoke and drink are also at increased risk of oral cancers.

Carcinogens contained in tobacco smoke have been found in cervical mucus, which perhaps explains the increased risk of cervical cancer in smokers. Cigarette smoking increases the incidence of duodenal ulcers and slows their healing. Studies have shown that failure to quit smoking may prevent ulcer healing even in patients who are otherwise appropriately treated. Alcohol is associated with gastritis and gastric ulcer disease, but not with duodenal ulcer disease.

Osteoporotic hip fractures are more prevalent in thin women who smoke and in alcoholics. The biologic explanation for these epidemiological findings is uncertain. Other important risk factors include advanced age, female sex, and white race.

Primary and Secondary Prevention of Specific Illnesses

DIRECTIONS: Each question below contains five suggested responses. Select the **one best** response to each question.

329. Correct statements concerning fluoridation of drinking water include all the following EXCEPT

(A) fluoridation of drinking water reduces caries by about 50 percent
(B) the advisability of fluoridation is still controversial among dental public health experts
(C) the optimum concentration of fluoride in public drinking water depends on the average daily air temperature of the community served
(D) fluorosis, a white or brown discoloration of the teeth from too much fluoride, often occurs if fluoride intake exceeds 4 to 8 mg per 24 h
(E) most people cannot taste fluoride at concentrations of 1 part per million (ppm)

330. True statements regarding type B *Haemophilus influenzae* include all the following EXCEPT

(A) it is a more important cause of mortality in children than in adults
(B) conjugated polysaccharide vaccine should be given to children beginning at 2 months of age
(C) it is the most common cause of acute otitis media in children
(D) it is the major cause of acute epiglottitis
(E) it is resistant to ampicillin in over 15 percent of cases

331. Which of the following prenatal screening tests is recommended for all pregnant women?

(A) Hemoglobin electrophoresis
(B) Hepatitis B surface antigen
(C) HIV antibody
(D) Ultrasound
(E) None of the above

332. Which of the following statements concerning the ELISA test for the detection of antibodies to the human immuno-deficiency virus (HIV) is true?

(A) Licensed kits, used under optimal conditions, have about a 50 percent sensitivity and specificity
(B) False negative results can occur in the first 12 weeks after infection
(C) The ELISA test has a high positive predictive value even in low-risk populations
(D) A person with one positive ELISA test should be told that he or she is infected with HIV
(E) None of the above

333. Correct statements concerning dietary iron and anemia include all the following EXCEPT

(A) serum ferritin and transferrin saturation should be obtained when performing primary screening for iron-deficiency anemia
(B) hemoglobin levels below those considered normal for pregnancy have been associated with infants of low birth weight
(C) the most common cause of anemia in the U.S. is iron deficiency
(D) iron deficiency anemia occurs most frequently in young children, women of reproductive age, and the elderly
(E) iron-rich foods include lean meats and whole grain products

334. True statements regarding the use of electrocardiography (ECG) as a screening tool for coronary artery disease (CAD) include all the following EXCEPT

(A) an exercise ECG is an appropriate screening test for sedentary or high-risk males over age 40 who are planning to begin a vigorous exercise program

(B) exercise ECG screening is recommended for adolescents planning on playing competitive athletics

(C) an exercise ECG is a more sensitive and specific screening test than a resting ECG

(D) false positive ECG results are not uncommon in healthy persons

(E) screening of asymptomatic persons is not recommended as an effective strategy to decrease the risk of CAD

335. All the following statements regarding screening for thyroid disease are true EXCEPT

(A) all neonates should be screened for congenital hypothyroidism

(B) although women are at an increased risk for thyroid cancer, ultrasound screening examinations are recommended only for those women with symptoms

(C) neck palpation is an accurate method to detect thyroid disease

(D) it is prudent to screen asymptomatic patients with a history of receiving upper-body irradiation during their childhood

(E) serum levels of thyroid hormones characteristic of thyroid disease are often influenced by a variety of biological factors

336. Correct statements regarding hepatitis B include all the following EXCEPT

(A) vertical transmission is a major public health problem in Asia
(B) vertical transmission can be prevented by hepatitis B immune globulin and hepatitis B vaccine
(C) persons working in dialysis units are at particularly high risk of occupational exposure
(D) transmission is primarily via the fecal-oral route in the U.S.
(E) chronic carriers are at increased risk of hepatocellular carcinoma

337. Prevention and control of infection in a hospital setting include all the following EXCEPT

(A) retrospective surveillance of nosocomial infections of patients
(B) isolation of patients with communicable disease
(C) employment of practitioners of infection control
(D) investigation of epidemic and endemic infections
(E) a physician who serves as hospital epidemiologist

338. Which of the following statements about the risks and benefits of postmenopausal hormonal replacement therapy is true?

(A) The increased risk of endometrial cancer is especially high among women using combination preparations (estrogen and progestin)
(B) The main potential benefit is a reduced risk of hip fracture
(C) Most studies have shown a reduced risk of breast cancer among women using estrogen-only preparations
(D) Most studies have shown a beneficial effect on mortality from coronary heart disease
(E) There is a slightly increased risk of pulmonary embolism

339. The case fatality rate of cholera is currently less than 1 percent. Major factors responsible for this low case fatality rate include

(A) treatment with tetracycline or other antibiotics
(B) mass immunization in endemic regions
(C) widespread use of intravenous hydration
(D) chlorination of water supplies in endemic regions
(E) none of the above

340. Immunization of preschool children with diphtheria toxoid results in

(A) protection against the diphtheria carrier state
(B) lifelong immunity against diphtheria
(C) detectable antitoxin for about 10 years
(D) frequent adverse reactions
(E) protection against infection of the respiratory tract by *Corynebacterium diphtheriae*

341. Epidemics of typhus fever have been associated with war and famine for several centuries. What factor was most important in the control of such epidemics following the end of World War II?

(A) Eradication of *Anopheles* mosquitoes
(B) Improved sanitation practices
(C) Improved methods for handling food supplies
(D) Disinfestation by use of DDT
(E) Mass therapy with antibiotics

342. The administration of a single injection of live attenuated measles vaccine results in

(A) seroconversion in 95 percent of susceptible children
(B) the induction of active immunity that lasts less than 5 years
(C) postimmunization encephalitis in 0.1 percent of recipients
(D) subacute sclerosing panencephalitis in 0.017 percent of recipients
(E) no significant risk to children with leukemia

343. Preventive treatment with isoniazid (isonicotinic acid hydrazide) is recommended for all the following groups EXCEPT

(A) young adults in whom a positive tuberculin test is demonstrated
(B) children under age 3 in whom a positive tuberculin test is demonstrated
(C) all members of a household in which one member has an active case of tuberculosis
(D) children with atypical mycobacterial infection
(E) nursing mothers with positive tuberculin skin tests

344. Passive immunization is the major means of prevention of which of the following diseases?

(A) Influenza
(B) German measles
(C) Mumps
(D) Viral hepatitis type A
(E) None of the above

345. Reasons to treat gonorrhea with oral tetracycline 500 mg qid for 7 days—rather than with oral ampicillin 3.5 g plus oral probenecid 1 g taken at one time—include

(A) lower frequency of side effects
(B) better coverage of *Chlamydia trachomatis*
(C) greater safety in case of pregnancy
(D) enhanced compliance
(E) none of the above

346. All the following statements concerning rotavirus are correct EXCEPT

(A) it is the most common cause of diarrhea in the U.S.
(B) it is probably spread via the fecal-oral route
(C) it is most common in the summer months in temperate climates
(D) adults with an infection may be asymptomatic
(E) viral shedding continues for at least 2 days after the diarrhea stops

347. All the following statements concerning tuberculosis (TB) are correct EXCEPT

(A) public health departments do not require case reporting of children with positive reactions to tuberculin purified protein derivative (PPD) if antibiotic treatment is initiated
(B) infants and children with primary TB are generally not infectious
(C) BCG vaccination has been shown to protect against TB meningitis and disseminated disease in children less than 5 years of age
(D) prevalence of infection detected by tuberculin testing increases with age
(E) isoniazid treatment is recommended for infected persons under 35 years of age

348. Correct statements about hepatitis B virus include all the following EXCEPT

(A) the incubation period for hepatitis B is longer than that for hepatitis A
(B) prevention of hepatitis B infection can be accomplished by means of hyperimmune globulin or vaccine
(C) specific diagnostic tests are not available for hepatitis B
(D) hepatitis B virus may persist in the blood for years
(E) the recombinant vaccine uses hepatitis B surface antigen

349. Prevention of human brucellosis depends on

(A) pasteurization of dairy products derived from goats, sheep, or cows
(B) treatment of human cases
(C) control of the insect vector
(D) immunization of farmers and slaughterhouse workers
(E) none of the above

350. Influenza vaccine is generally recommended for which of the following groups?

(A) All persons over 55 years of age
(B) School-age children
(C) All persons with severe pulmonary disorders regardless of age
(D) Pregnant women
(E) None of the above

351. Often, visual disturbances and sore throat are the first symptoms in cases of botulism. Other characteristics of botulism are described by all the following statements EXCEPT

(A) in the U.S. most cases result from inadequate processing of home-canned foods
(B) the incubation period is usually 12 to 36 h
(C) toxins produced by *Clostridium botulinum* are destroyed by boiling
(D) death is most often the result of the effect of the toxin on the myocardium
(E) it should be treated with antitoxin

352. Which of the following statements regarding herpes simplex virus, type 2 (HSV-2), is correct?

(A) Infections with HSV-2 are almost always symptomatic
(B) Transmission from mother to infant is generally transplacental
(C) HSV infection is an early sign of the acquired immunodeficiency syndrome
(D) Neonates with cutaneous disease should receive antiviral therapy regardless of whether there is evidence of dissemination
(E) None of the above

353. Which of the following statements about rubella (German measles) is correct?

(A) Significant subscapular and axillary lymphadenopathy is common
(B) The vaccine incorporates a killed virus
(C) Rubella immunization should be routinely offered to potentially susceptible postpubertal women
(D) Exposure to rubella early in pregnancy usually does not affect the fetus
(E) Therapy with corticosteroids is not a contraindication to immunization

354. Effective means of preventing trichinosis in humans include

(A) cooking pork and pork products to ensure that all parts of the meat reach a temperature of at least 40°C (104° F)
(B) attention to proper disposal of hog feces
(C) prohibiting the marketing of garbage-fed hogs
(D) skin testing of hogs with *Trichinella* antigen prior to slaughter
(E) none of the above

355. True statements about Lyme disease include

(A) it is caused by an arthropod-borne virus (arbovirus)
(B) it is associated with a characteristic skin rash, called erythema marginatum centrificum (EMC)
(C) it occurs primarily in the Rocky Mountain states of the U.S.
(D) it may involve the heart and the central nervous system, as well as joints
(E) none of the above

356. Diseases that are transmitted chiefly from person to person include

(A) California encephalitis
(B) St. Louis encephalitis
(C) lymphocytic choriomeningitis
(D) meningococcal meningitis
(E) none of the above

357. In the U.S. exfoliative cytology is the most commonly used test for detection of cancer of the

(A) skin
(B) breast
(C) stomach
(D) colon
(E) cervix

358. Major risk factors for coronary artery disease include all the following EXCEPT

(A) an elevated low-density lipoprotein (LDL) level
(B) an elevated high-density lipoprotein (HDL) level
(C) hypertension
(D) cigarette smoking
(E) male sex

359. Which of the following statements about the treatment of hypertension is true?

(A) Treating hypertension has been shown to reduce the incidence of stroke

(B) Treating mild-to-moderate hypertension has been shown to reduce the incidence of coronary heart disease

(C) Most persons with hypertension in the U.S. are not aware that they have high blood pressure

(D) No study has ever demonstrated a benefit from treating hypertension in men

(E) No study has ever demonstrated a benefit from treating hypertension in women

360. All the following techniques are considered useful in screening for cancer in asymptomatic persons EXCEPT

(A) breast self-examination in a 45-year-old woman

(B) mammography in a 45-year-old woman

(C) mammography in a 55-year-old woman

(D) Pap smear in a 55-year-old female smoker

(E) chest radiography in a 55-year-old male smoker

361. True statements regarding blood lipoproteins include all the following EXCEPT

(A) mean levels of total serum cholesterol of immigrants rapidly approach those of the adopted country, whether higher or lower than the country of origin

(B) average levels of total serum cholesterol differ widely for populations of school-age children

(C) associations are consistently strong between mean population levels of total serum cholesterol and measured incidence of coronary artery disease

(D) large-scale trials have failed to demonstrate the feasibility of lowering blood cholesterol through dietary changes

(E) in the U.S., over the past 20 years there has probably been a significant decrease in the mean level of total serum cholesterol

362. All the following are dietary determinants of plasma lipid levels EXCEPT

(A) alcohol
(B) total calories
(C) cholesterol
(D) saturated fat
(E) vitamin E

363. Use of postmenopausal estrogens has been consistently associated with

(A) an increased risk of endometrial cancer
(B) a decreased risk of breast cancer
(C) an increased risk of osteoporotic fractures
(D) an increased risk of coronary heart disease
(E) an increased incidence of liver cancer

364. Which of the following statements about blood pressure is true?

(A) Isolated systolic hypertension is defined as a systolic blood pressure above 200 mmHg with a normal diastolic blood pressure
(B) Isolated systolic hypertension is a risk factor for stroke
(C) Diastolic blood pressure is a more important predictor of incidence of coronary heart disease than is systolic blood pressure
(D) The prevalence of isolated systolic hypertension increases with age in men but not in women
(E) The prevalence of isolated systolic hypertension peaks between ages 60 and 70

365. Which of the following statements about inflammatory bowel disease is true?

(A) The incidence of ulcerative colitis is lower in Jews
(B) Total colectomy to prevent malignancy is recommended for all persons who have had ulcerative colitis for more than 20 years
(C) The incidence of Crohn's disease is increased in Jews
(D) Total colectomy to prevent malignancy is recommended for all persons who have had Crohn's disease of the colon for more than 20 years
(E) Both Crohn's disease and ulcerative colitis are more common in men than in women

366. The prognosis for patients with coronary artery disease is related to all the following EXCEPT

(A) serum cholesterol level
(B) left ventricular function
(C) family history of heart disease
(D) degree of coronary artery stenosis
(E) severity of ischemia

367. The major environmental source of lead absorbed in the human blood stream in adults is

(A) air
(B) water
(C) lead-based paint
(D) food
(E) none of the above

368. Inherent difficulties in understanding and preventing occupational disease and injury include all the following EXCEPT

(A) interventions needed to decrease exposure to known hazards are often expensive
(B) most U.S. physicians lack knowledge about occupational medicine
(C) even when an association between a chemical exposure and a disease is clearly documented, it may be difficult to establish an etiological relationship in an individual
(D) the study of adverse effects of exposure on exposed workers is usually complex and costly
(E) U.S. regulatory agencies have not established testing guidelines

369. The key factors involved in the prevention of back injuries include all the following EXCEPT

(A) the prevention of the first injury, since subsequent injuries are more likely to occur
(B) the elimination or decrease of awkward trunk postures and prolonged sitting
(C) the development of weight-lifting limits adjusted for the age and physical condition of workers
(D) the requirement of preemployment radiographs of the lumbosacral spine
(E) mechanical lifting devices

370. Permissible exposure limits (PELs) are used by industries and government agencies to describe the allowable amount of a toxic chemical to which persons may be occupationally exposed. PELs are correctly described by which of the following statements?

(A) They are based on consideration of the acute and long-term health effects of hazardous substances
(B) They have been established for most chemicals in use by industry
(C) Employers are not responsible for surveying and sampling for chemical exposure
(D) They do not require a monitoring system to evaluate the levels of chemicals in the worker's environment
(E) None of the above

371. Several nonmodifiable individual risk factors—such as age, gender, and family history—are associated with the occurrence of many psychiatric disorders. All the following statements regarding these factors are true EXCEPT

(A) after a peak among 18- to 35-year-old persons, rates of depression and anxiety decline in older persons
(B) before puberty males have more psychopathology than do females
(C) males have higher rates of depression and phobias
(D) in first-degree relatives of persons with depression, the rate of depression is twice normal
(E) there is a genetic vulnerability to alcoholism

372. Infants born to mothers addicted to cocaine are at increased risk for which of the following problems?

(A) Micrognathia
(B) Cardiac defects
(C) Minor joint and limb abnormalities
(D) Seizures
(E) Excessive birth weight

373. Characteristic signs or symptoms of kwashiorkor include all the following EXCEPT

(A) hypoalbuminemia
(B) loss of subcutaneous fat
(C) edema
(D) diarrhea
(E) ulcerated skin lesions

374. Which of the following statements about the use of nicotine-containing chewing gum to help cigarette smokers quit smoking is true?

(A) It most successful in persons who are not addicted to nicotine
(B) It is most successful in persons with low levels of addiction to nicotine
(C) It is most successful in persons with moderate levels of addiction to nicotine
(D) It is most successful in persons with high levels of addiction to nicotine
(E) Its success is unrelated to the degree of nicotine addiction

375. True statements regarding herpes simplex virus (HSV) include all the following EXCEPT

(A) HSV-1 ultimately infects most of the human race
(B) condoms are probably more effective in preventing HIV than HSV-2 transmission
(C) most neonatal HSV is seen following vaginal delivery in symptomatic mothers
(D) frequent handwashing by hospital staff helps to decrease transmission of HSV
(E) diagnosis of HSV can be made by visual inspection of skin lesions as well as by viral culture

DIRECTIONS: Each group of questions below consists of lettered headings followed by a set of numbered items. For each numbered item select the **one** lettered heading with which it is **most** closely associated. Each lettered heading may be used **once, more than once, or not at all.**

Questions 376–379

Match each set of symptoms and signs with the dietary deficiency.

(A) Vitamin A deficiency
(B) Thiamine deficiency
(C) Vitamin C deficiency
(D) Vitamin D deficiency
(E) Niacin deficiency

376. Petechiae, sore gums, hematuria, and bone or joint pain

377. Dermatitis, diarrhea, and delirium

378. Edema, neuropathy, and myocardial failure

379. Conjunctival xerosis, hyperkeratosis, and keratomalacia

Questions 380–384

For each preventive health measure or concern, select the age range with which it is associated.

(A) Birth to 18 months
(B) Ages 2 to 6
(C) Ages 7 to 12
(D) Ages 13 to 18

380. Initial blood pressure screening

381. Initial dental visit

382. Tetanus-diphtheria (Td) booster

383. Routine blood testing

384. Suicide as a leading cause of death

Questions 385–388

Match each of the descriptions below with the correct worm.

(A) *Necator americanus* (hookworm)
(B) *Ascaris lumbricoides* (roundworm)
(C) *Strongyloides stercoralis*
(D) *Taenia solium* (pork tapeworm)
(E) *Trichuris trichiura* (whipworm)

385. Infection follows ingestion of embryonated eggs, which mature into larvae in the intestine, then migrate to the lungs to mature further

386. Infection of man by this worm in the larval stage is termed *cysticercosis*

387. Intestinal autoinfection may lead to increasing worm burden and dissemination

388. Acquired when infective larvae penetrate the skin; main symptoms are due to iron deficiency

Questions 389–392

For each description below, match the appropriate arthropod parasite.

(A) *Sarcoptes scabiei*
(B) *Pediculus humanus capitis*
(C) *Pediculus humanus corporis*
(D) *Phthirius pubis*
(E) None of the above

389. Vector for epidemic typhus and relapsing fever

390. Epidemics in school children; best treated with a 1% permethrin preparation

391. Vector for Lyme disease

392. Burrows under the skin

Questions 393–396

Match the effect of deficiency to the proper mineral.

(A) Fluorine
(B) Copper
(C) Zinc
(D) Sodium
(E) Calcium

393. Poor mineralization of bones and teeth; osteoporosis

394. Nausea; diarrhea; muscle cramps; dehydration

395. Tendency to dental caries

396. Dwarfism; hepatosplenomegaly; poor wound healing

Questions 397–401

Match the following ethnic groups with the disease for which it would be most appropriate to institute a screening program.

(A) Alpha thalassemia
(B) Beta thalassemia
(C) Cystic fibrosis
(D) Hemophilia
(E) Tay-Sachs disease

397. Italians

398. Chinese

399. Ashkenazic Jews

400. Greeks

401. Germans

Questions 402–405

Match the disease with the causative agent.

(A) *Neisseria gonorrhoeae*
(B) *Giardia lamblia*
(C) Human papillomavirus (HPV)
(D) Human immunodeficiency virus (HIV)
(E) Group B streptococcus

402. Enteritis

403. Cervical neoplasia

404. Non-Hodgkin's lymphoma

405. Urethritis

Questions 406–409

For each disease, choose the most effective or principal means of control.

(A) Rat control
(B) Sanitation
(C) Immunization
(D) Vector control
(E) None of the above

406. AIDS

407. St. Louis encephalitis

408. Typhoid fever

409. Tetanus

Questions 410–413

Match the following.

(A) Hemolytic anemia in premature infants
(B) Hemorrhagic disease of the newborn
(C) Wound healing
(D) Rickets
(E) Polyneuritis

410. Vitamin C

411. Vitamin E

412. Vitamin D

413. Vitamin K

Questions 414–417

For each disease, indicate the material in which the infectious agent is transmitted from the infected host.

(A) Conjunctival exudate
(B) Lesion exudate
(C) Blood
(D) Respiratory secretions
(E) Feces

414. Syphilis

415. Shigellosis

416. Pertussis

417. Trachoma

Questions 418–421

Match each infection below with the intermediate host involved in transmission.

(A) Snail
(B) Swine
(C) Fish
(D) Crab
(E) Dog

418. Paragonimiasis (lung fluke disease)

419. Diphyllobothriasis

420. Toxocariasis (visceral larva migrans)

421. Cysticercosis

Questions 422–425

Select the reservoir for each of the diseases below.

(A) Cattle
(B) Humans
(C) Rodents
(D) Ticks
(E) Mosquitoes
(F) None of the above

422. Candidiasis

423. Plague

424. Brucellosis

425. Enterobiasis

Primary and Secondary Prevention of Specific Illnesses

Answers

329. The answer is B. *(Behrman, 14/e, p 110. Last, Maxcy-Rosenau, 13/e, pp 627–628.)* Because of the consistent effectiveness of fluoride in reducing dental caries by about 50 percent, its use is now widely accepted among public health professionals. Controversy surrounding fluoridation is political, not scientific. The optimum concentration of fluoride in drinking water decreases with increasing mean air temperature because people drink more water when it is hotter.

330. The answer is C. *(Last, Maxcy-Rosenau, 13/e, pp 85–87, 207–209.)* Type B *Haemophilus influenzae* is by far the most virulent type and accounts for almost all cases of invasive disease. (Remember: B is for bad.) The most important of these diseases are meningitis, epiglottitis, pneumonia, and periorbital or facial cellulitis, and their occurrence is mainly in children. Previous vaccines were not effective in children under 18 months of age. However, a new vaccine made of capsular polysaccharide conjugated with diphtheria toxoid can be given to children beginning at 2 months of age. *H. influenzae* is the second most common cause of acute otitis media in children (after pneumococcus), but most cases are due to nontypable strains, rather than to type B. Because ampicillin resistance is increasingly common, life-threatening *H. influenzae* infections should be initially treated with both ampicillin and chloramphenicol, or with one of the newer cephalosporins, such as cefotaxime or ceftriaxone.

331. The answer is B. *(USPS Task Force, pp lvi-lvii, 121–124, 139–146, 201–208, 225–232.)* Universal screening for hepatitis B surface antigen (HBsAg) in pregnant women is based on evidence that early treatment of the newborn with hepatitis B immune globulin and subsequent vaccination is 85 to 95 percent effective in preventing development of the chronic carrier state in infants born to HBsAg-positive mothers. Screening only high-risk groups misses 35 to 65 percent of chronic carriers, presumably because of lack of information about maternal substance abuse and sexual habits. Since the test and treatment are both efficacious and relatively inexpensive, and there is a large at-risk population, routine screening is recommended. In populations where hepatitis B is endemic (e.g., Alaskan natives, Pacific islanders), universal vaccination with hepatitis B vaccine may be more practical.

Currently, HIV testing is recommended only for mothers identified as high-risk, although this recommendation could change as the AIDS epidemic spreads and evidence for the efficacy of early treatment of infants increases. Hemoglobin electrophoresis is only recommended for people at high risk for sickle cell anemia or thalassemia. Ultrasound is recommended for women with either uncertain menstrual histories or risk factors for intrauterine growth retardation.

332. The answer is B. *(USPS Task Force, pp 139–146.)* Commercially licensed ELISA kits for HIV detection have a sensitivity and specificity of 99 percent when used under optimal conditions. In reality, more false positives and false negatives probably occur. In the first 12 weeks of infection with HIV, antibodies may not have reached detectable levels; thus an ELISA test during this time may be falsely negative. Infected persons who are in this "window" period can probably transmit the disease. In low-risk populations even highly sensitive and specific tests have low positive predictive values. Thus screening of high-risk populations is much more likely to be beneficial than screening of low-risk populations. False positive results can be caused by nonspecific serologic reactions in persons with immunologic disturbances, as well as in persons with a history of multiple blood transfusions. Repeat ELISA tests are required for all positive first ELISAs in order to reduce the false positive rate. A reactive (positive) ELISA in sequential tests has a specificity of 99.8 percent. It is then verified with another test, such as the Western blot, radioimmunoassays, or indirect immunofluorescence assays.

333. The answer is A. *(USPS Task Force, pp 163–165, 307–309.)* Routine screening is recommended for all infants and pregnant women. Hemoglobin concentration and hematocrit are the principal screening tests. Other tests are not suitable because they are relatively expensive and because of the low prevalence of iron deficiency in the general U.S. population. Besides low birth weight, prematurity and high perinatal mortality have also been associated with maternal hemoglobin levels below those considered normal for pregnancy. The prevalence of iron deficiency has decreased in children recently, but it is still estimated to be about 3 percent for children from 1 to 5 years of age. Other groups with an elevated risk for anemia include African-Americans, persons of low socioeconomic status, and some immigrants. Lima beans, soybeans, brussels sprouts, green peas, and green leafy vegetables are among other iron-rich foods.

334. The answer is B. *(USPS Task Force, pp 3–7.)* Along with sedentary or high-risk males over 40 years of age, anyone who would endanger public safety if she or he were to experience a sudden cardiac event (e.g., airline pilots) should also have a screening exercise ECG. Children, adolescents, and young adults without evidence of heart disease do not require routine exercise or resting ECG to participate in athletics. The difficulty with ECG screening is that it is an imperfect test. Many false positives occur in low-risk asymptomatic populations. The economic impact of screening the low-risk population would be enormous. Screening patients with two or more cardiac risk factors (serum cholesterol > 240 mg/dL, blood pressure > 160/90 mmHg, cigarette smoking, diabetes mellitus, family history of CAD before age 55 years) is recommended by some.

335. The answer is C. *(USPS Task Force, pp 105–109.)* Screening for congenital hypothyroidism is recommended for all neonates during the first week of life. Heel-prick specimens for T_4 and TSH should be obtained. Routine thyroid function testing is otherwise not recommended for asymptomatic children or adults, but should be considered for populations at increased risk, such as the elderly (especially women), persons with a family history of multiple endocrine neoplasia syndrome II, and those who have received upper-body irradiation during childhood. Screening tests for the detection of thyroid cancer include neck palpation to detect nodules and diagnostic procedures such as scintigraphy, ultrasonography, and fine-needle aspiration with cytology. Only neck palpation is recommended as a screening test for asymptomatic persons. The sensitivity and specificity of neck palpation vary with the technique of the examiner and the size of the mass. The presence of nonthyroidal illness can produce spuriously low levels of T_3 and T_4 ("sick euthyroid syndrome") or may raise TSH and T_4 levels. Also, psychiatric disease may produce transient increases in thyroid hormones that later return to normal during recovery. For these reasons, estimates of the sensitivity and specificity of thyroid function tests vary with the type of test and type of thyroid dysfunction being sought.

336. The answer is D. *(Benenson, 15/e, pp 200–207.)* In some areas of Southeast Asia, the prevalence of the hepatitis B carrier state is 20 percent or more. Vertical transmission from asymptomatic infected mothers to their infants is thought to be the major mode of perpetuation of the high endemic carrier rate because hepatitis B acquired in infancy is much more likely to result in chronic infection than is infection acquired later. Chronic carriers are important not only as reservoirs for hepatitis, but also because of their very high risk of hepatocellular carcinoma. For this reason it is essential to screen women for hepatitis B carriage during their pregnancy so that the infant can be given hepatitis B immune globulin and hepatitis B vaccine, which have been shown to be 90 percent effective at interrupting vertical transmission of the disease. In the United States, the infection is primarily transmitted horizontally through exposure to blood or blood products via either needles (e.g., in drug addicts, recipients of factor VIII concentrate, hospital workers) or mucous membranes (via sexual contact). Employees of dialysis centers are among those at highest risk. The fecal-oral route is not an important route of transmission of hepatitis B, although it is for hepatitis A.

337. The answer is A. *(Last, Maxcy-Rosenau, 13/e, pp 206–207.)* Prospective surveillance programs are much more valuable in determining if nosocomial infections have occurred than retrospective surveillance. They are also important in selecting the appropriate intervention. Surveillance based on discharge diagnoses is flawed because of underreporting and failure to use standard criteria for diagnosis. Guidelines for instrumentation of patients are also important in controlling infections. Nonphysician practitioners of infection control usually coordinate the surveillance and control programs. A CDC study in the mid-70s found that the presence of at least one full-time infection-control nurse for every 250 beds significantly improved the effectiveness of infection-control programs. A physician epidemiologist who takes responsibility for the infection-control program is essential. The physician serves as supervisor to infection-control practitioners, provides liaison with other medical staff, provides advice about various epidemiological aspects of infection control, and advises the hospital medical staff and administration regarding clinical implications of care practices, infection problems, and prevention and control measures.

338. The answer is D. *(Wilson, 12/e, p 1793.)* Most authorities believe that adding a progestin will reduce the risk of endometrial cancer associated with estrogen-only preparations. The effects on coronary heart disease, which is the leading cause of mortality in women, are the most

important. Unlike oral contraceptives, there is no effect of postmenopausal hormonal replacement therapy on pulmonary embolism. There
may be a slightly increased risk of breast cancer.

339. The answer is A. *(Benenson, 15/e, pp 89–94.)* Antibiotics and oral
fluid therapy have been the major factors in reducing the case fatality
rate of cholera. Treatment of cholera with tetracycline reduces the volume and duration of diarrhea and thus reduces the need for intravenous
administration of fluids. Glucose-electrolyte solutions for oral administration not only have been shown to be well absorbed and capable of
maintaining fluid and electrolyte balance but also have reduced the need
for intravenous fluid therapy. An effective cholera vaccine has not yet
been developed. In any case, vaccination and chlorination would be
expected to reduce the incidence, not the case fatality rate.

340. The answer is C. *(Benenson, 15/e, pp 138–142.)* Diphtheria toxoid, alone or in combination with pertussis vaccine and tetanus toxoid
(DPT), induces protective levels of antitoxin that persist for about 10
years. Boosters are required every 10 years after completion of primary
immunization in order to maintain protective concentration of antibody.
Antitoxin antibodies do not prevent infection of the respiratory tract
with *C. diphtheriae* and do not prevent the development of the carrier
state. The antibodies are directed against the exotoxin produced by the
bacteria, not against the bacteria themselves. Adverse reactions from
the toxoid are very infrequent in infants and young children but are
more common in adults; therefore, the administration of a reduced dose
of toxoid is recommended for children over 6 years of age and adults.
The reduced dose is symbolized by a lower case *d*. It is usually combined with tetanus toxoid as a Td.

341. The answer is D. *(Benenson, 15/e, pp 474–479.)* The infectious
agent for epidemic forms of typhus fever is *Rickettsia prowazecki*,
which is transmitted from person to person by the human body louse,
Pediculus humanus corporis. Disruptions of social and economic institutions by war, famine, or natural catastrophes are associated with declining standards of personal hygiene and spread of lice. Even before
social and economic recovery after World War II, epidemic typhus was
controlled by mass application of DDT powder. This insecticide killed
the body lice; thus the transmission cycle was interrupted. Effective
antibiotic therapy with chloramphenicol and tetracycline was not available until the early 1950s. *Anopheles* mosquitoes are vectors in the
transmission of malaria, not typhus.

342. The answer is A. *(Benenson, 15/e, pp 269–275.)* The injection of live attenuated measles vaccine induces protective antibodies in 95 percent of susceptible children; this seroconversion, or development of active immunity, persists for over 12 years. Postimmunization encephalitis is very rare (1 per 1 million doses) and subacute sclerosing panencephalitis has not been linked definitely to vaccine use. Leukemia and other conditions associated with immunosuppression are contraindications to the use of live measles vaccine because of the risk of developing severe or fatal giant-cell pneumonia.

343. The answer is D. *(Benenson, 15/e, pp 457–465.)* Preventive treatment is treatment of *inactive* tuberculosis—that is, tuberculosis without evidence of disease—and has as its objective the reduction of the incidence of active tuberculosis. Preventive treatment with isoniazid, or isonicotinic acid hydrazide (INH), is recommended for children and young adults whose tuberculin tests are positive, for those who have had contact with persons who have recently converted to tuberculin positivity, and for immunosuppressed persons whose tuberculin tests are positive. Because of the risk of INH-associated hepatitis, preventive treatment with INH is no longer routinely recommended for adults over age 35 and is not recommended for prevention of tuberculosis caused by atypical mycobacteria. Breast feeding is not a contraindication to INH. In a risk-benefit analysis to assess the potential effectiveness of INH, consideration should be given to the high susceptibility to infection of children under 3 years of age, of adolescents, and of young adults.

344. The answer is D. *(Benenson, 15/e, pp 197–200, 224–229, 293–296, 376–380.)* Passive immunization is the provision of antibodies that are already formed rather than of antigens, which are used for active immunization. For example, viral hepatitis type A infection can be prevented by the administration of immune serum globulin. German measles, mumps, and influenza are best prevented by active immunization with vaccines.

345. The answer is B. *(Benenson, 15/e, pp 185–188.)* Both tetracycline 500 mg qid for a week and ampicillin 3.5 g plus probenecid 1 g taken at one time are effective in eradicating non-penicillinase-producing *Neisseria gonorrhoeae*. The single dose therapy has the advantages of improved compliance and infrequent side effects. However, because up to 45 percent of patients with gonorrhea have coexisting chlamydial infection, tetracycline should be considered, in spite of its less convenient dosage schedule and tendency to cause mild gastrointestinal discomfort. (These problems are less severe with doxycycline, but doxycycline is considerably more expensive.) In addition, many authorities recommend combining the treatments to get the benefits of both. Pregnancy is a contraindication to treatment with tetracycline because of possible effects on the developing teeth.

346. The answer is C. *(Behrman, 14/e, pp 664, 831–832. Benenson, 15/e, pp 178–180.)* Rotavirus is the most common agent responsible for diarrhea in infants throughout the world. It causes 1,000,000 deaths per year worldwide and accounts for approximately 70,000 hospitalizations in the U.S. Children under 2 years of age are the most commonly infected population. Hospitals often have epidemics, as do day-care centers. Rotavirus infections are most common in the winter in temperate climates, with epidemics spreading from west to east across the U.S. Adults may acquire an infection from an infected infant or as traveler's diarrhea. Sanitary disposal of diapers is an extremely important control measure. Patients are able to transmit the disease during viral shedding, which can last longer than 30 days in immunocompromised persons.

347. The answer is A. *(Behrman, 14/e, pp 763–772. Benenson, 15/e, pp 457–465.)* All positive PPDs should be reported to public health officials. Primary infection with tubercle bacilli usually occurs following inhalation of airborne droplets containing the microorganism. Although infected adults may produce airborne droplets with coughing, sneezing, or singing, infants and children with primary TB may not cough. Children (3 to 15 years) usually have a brief, asymptomatic primary pulmonary infection. BCG vaccination is valuable in high-risk populations, but because the risk of infection is low in most parts of the U.S., BCG is not routinely used. It may be considered for children with negative PPDs who cannot be placed on preventive isoniazid therapy and who have continuous exposure to persons with active disease. BCG is contraindicated for persons with symptomatic HIV infection. Isoniazid treatment has been shown to prevent the progression of latent disease to clinical disease in a high percentage of persons. However, because there is an increased risk of isoniazid-associated hepatitis in older persons, it is not routinely recommended for infected persons older than 35 years. In those infected persons younger than 35 years, isoniazid preventive treatment is recommended, usually in combination with rifampin with or without pyrazinamide, for at least 6 months.

348. The answer is C. *(Benenson, 15/e, pp 200–207.)* Hepatitis B virus (HBV) infection has an incubation period of 6 weeks to 6 months, compared with 2 to 6 weeks for infections caused by hepatitis A virus (HAV). Specific diagnosis of HBV infection can be made by the detection of hepatitis B surface antigen (HBsAg) in the blood during the acute stage of the infection or by detecting antibodies to a variety of antigens of HBV in the convalescent stage. HBsAg may persist in the blood for many years: the chronic carrier state develops in 10 percent of HBV infections in adults. Chronic carriage of HBsAg is associated with a significantly increased risk of chronic hepatitis, cirrhosis, and hepatocellular carcinoma. Hepatitis B immune globulin (HBIG), a preparation of immune globulin containing high titers of anti-HBs, is an effective means of preventing infection if administered within 72 h after exposure to HBV. Vaccines made from either highly purified HBsAg derived from plasma of healthy chronic carriers or from HBsAg produced by genetically engineered bacteria have been shown to be highly effective in preventing HBV infection. Administration of HBIG followed by three doses of vaccine is 90 percent effective in preventing vertical (mother-to-baby) transmission.

349. The answer is A. *(Benenson, 15/e, pp 66–68.)* Prevention of human brucellosis depends on pasteurization of dairy products from cows, goats, and sheep; education of farmers and workers in the livestock industry as to dangers of infected animals; and care in handling products from aborted animals. There is no insect vector. No vaccine for human use is available. Since person-to-person transmission does not occur, treatment of individual cases will not control spread of brucellosis.

350. The answer is C. *(Benenson, 15/e, pp 224–229.)* Influenza vaccine is not recommended for routine use in the entire population because current vaccines produce immunity lasting only 1 to 2 years and are only 60 to 70 percent effective. Periodic changes in the viral antigens also contribute to absence of long-term efficacy of vaccines. High-risk groups include all persons over 65 years of age, persons with chronic heart and lung conditions, and persons with other chronic diseases such as diabetes, neuromuscular disorders, and renal failure. Pregnant women have not been shown to be at increased risk of excess morbidity or mortality during recent epidemics. Routine immunization of school children is not recommended with the current vaccines even though school-age children are the major age group involved in the transmission of influenza in the community. If safe, effective vaccines with long-lasting immunity are developed, school children will be the major target group.

351. The answer is D. *(Benenson, 15/e, pp 61–66.)* Botulism is an intoxication by the exotoxin produced by *Clostridium botulinum,* a gram-positive, spore-forming bacterium. The incubation period is usually 12 to 36 h. In the U.S. most cases are associated with ingestion of improperly home-canned vegetables, fish, and fruits, especially foods that are slightly acidic. The toxin is destroyed by boiling for at least 3 min, but higher temperatures are needed to kill the spores. At inadequate temperatures, spores are not destroyed; they subsequently germinate and multiply under anaerobic conditions. Death is usually the consequence of respiratory paralysis or secondary infection. An antitoxin is available and is considered part of routine treatment.

352. The answer is D. *(Last, Maxcy-Rosenau, 13/e, pp 105–106, 142–144.)* HSV-2, the main cause of genital herpes, is currently epidemic in the U.S. Many infections are asymptomatic, which makes it difficult to prevent further spread. Infants acquire the infection from their mothers during vaginal delivery; for mothers with known active HSV-2 infections, caesarian delivery within 4 h of rupture of membranes is indicated. HSV-2 infection is not an early sign of AIDS; unlike infections such as *Pneumocystis carinii,* its occurrence does not suggest immunosuppression. However, infection with HSV-2, as with syphilis, has been linked to higher risks of HIV infection among homosexual men. Neonates with any signs of HSV infection should receive antiviral therapy; one of the goals is to prevent dissemination.

353. The answer is C. *(Behrman, 14/e, pp 520–523, 794–796.)* The retroauricular, posterior cervical, and postoccipital lymph nodes are most noticeably enlarged and tender. The rubella vaccine is a live-virus vaccine and should not be given to pregnant women. Antibody develops in approximately 98 percent of those vaccinated, but the duration of antibody is uncertain. To protect the fetus, it is important that girls have immunity to rubella before they reach child-bearing age. Rubella titers may also be drawn to determine antibody status. Rates of congenital infection following primary maternal infection range from 75 to 90 percent in the first trimester, 25 to 39 percent in the second trimester, and 24 to 53 percent in the third trimester. Manifestations of congenital rubella range from intrauterine and postnatal growth retardation to deafness and psychomotor retardation. Any immune deficiency state, severe febrile illness, hypersensitivity to vaccine components, and therapy with antimetabolites, corticosteroids and corticosteroid-like substances are all considered contraindications to immunization with live virus.

354. The answer is C. *(Benenson, 15/e, pp 446–448. Last, Maxcy-Rosenau, 13/e, pp 269–270.)* Infection of hogs with nematodes of the genus *Trichinella* can be prevented by ensuring that all garbage and offal fed to the hogs are heat-treated to destroy the cysts or, preferably, by using feed devoid of animal meat, such as grain. Prohibition of marketing of garbage-fed hogs is easier to enforce than inspection to ensure that all garbage is properly cooked. Thorough cooking of pork and pork products so that all the meat reaches at least 77°C (171°F) destroys the encysted larvae. Freezing pork also destroys the larvae if adequate time-temperature schedules are followed. The disease is transmitted by ingestion of larvae in skeletal muscle, not by hog feces.

355. The answer is D. *(Benenson, 15/e, pp 255–257.)* Lyme disease is caused by a spirochete, *Borrelia burgdorferi,* transmitted to humans by the bite of infected ticks. The name comes from the town (Old Lyme, Connecticut) from which the first cases were reported. There are endemic foci on the east coast from Massachusetts to Virginia, and in Wisconsin, Minnesota, California, and Oregon. The hallmark of the disease is the characteristic rash, which begins as a red papule (usually at the site of the tick bite) and slowly spreads outward in an advancing annular fashion. This lesion is called erythema chronicum migrans (ECM). Subsequently, joints (either acute or chronic arthritis), CNS (an aseptic meningitis or encephalitis), and heart (atrioventricular arrhythmias or myopericarditis) may be involved. These complications may be diminished by early treatment with tetracycline or penicillin.

356. The answer is D. *(Benenson, 15/e, pp 31–35, 257–259, 280–284.)* Meningococcal disease is transmitted by direct contact with droplets and discharges from infected cases and, more often, carriers. California encephalitis and St. Louis encephalitis are acute, inflammatory diseases in which the causative virus is mosquito-transmitted. Lymphocytic choriomeningitis is caused by an arenavirus acquired from contact with food or dust contaminated with urine, saliva, and feces of infected mice. Person-to-person transmission does not occur in these last three diseases.

357. The answer is E. *(Wilson, 12/e, pp 1585–1586.)* The efficacy of exfoliative cytology (Pap smear) in early identification of uterine and cervical cancer has been demonstrated. Mortality from cervical cancer has consistently declined following screening programs based on the Pap smear. Current recommendations are to perform the test every 3 years following three normal Pap smears in consecutive years in women 20 to 40 years of age. In women over 40, yearly checkups are recommended.

358. The answer is B. *(Wilson, 12/e, pp 995–996.)* The most important preventable risk factors for coronary artery disease (CAD) are hypercholesterolemia (especially an elevated LDL level), cigarette smoking, and hypertension. Of these three risk factors, however, evidence from randomized trials showing a reduction in CAD is available only for treatment of elevated cholesterol levels. An elevated HDL level is associated with a reduced risk of CAD. The death rate from ischemic heart disease is five times higher in white men ages 35 to 55 compared with white women of the same age.

359. The answer is A. *(Wyngaarden, 19/e, pp 253–269.)* Treating hypertension can reduce the incidence of stroke by up to 90 percent. Most persons with hypertension in the U.S. (70 percent) are aware of their condition. Treatment of hypertension appears to be equally efficacious in men and women.

360. The answer is E. *(Last, Maxcy-Rosenau, 13/e, pp 822–825.)* The purpose of a cancer screening technique is to detect the disease at an asymptomatic phase. This is helpful only if early treatment is more effective than later treatment. Detection of lung cancer with radiography in asymptomatic smokers does not meet this requirement.

361. The answer is D. *(Last, 13/e, pp 827–840.)* The Multiple Risk Factor Intervention Trial and the National Diet-Heart Study found blood cholesterol can be lowered safely with dietary changes. Some of the dietary changes that have occurred over the past 20 years in some populations include a decrease in saturated fatty acids and cholesterol intake, which is associated with a decrease in serum cholesterol and a decrease in coronary artery disease. Japanese who immigrated to the U.S. became taller, heavier, more obese, and more sedentary than their counterparts in Japan. They eat more saturated fatty acids and cholesterol, meats, and dairy products and eat less complex carbohydrates.

Thus they develop higher rates of coronary artery disease within a generation.

362. The answer is E. *(Wilson, 12/e, pp 440–441, 998.)* Many patients with hypercholesterolemia can lower their plasma cholesterol levels by reducing the intake of total calories, saturated fat, cholesterol, and alcohol; however, dietary changes, unless they are severe, do not usually lower plasma cholesterol levels by more than 10 to 20 percent. In low-to-moderate quantities (about two drinks per day) alcohol increases the high-density lipoprotein levels (i.e., has a beneficial effect), whereas at higher doses it increases low-density lipoprotein levels (i.e., has a harmful effect). Vitamin E levels in serum are affected by lipid levels; however, the reverse is not true.

363. The answer is A. *(Wyngaarden, 19/e, p 1375.)* Postmenopausal estrogens (PME) are commonly prescribed for the relief of menopausal symptoms (such as hot flashes) and for the prevention of postmenopausal osteoporosis. They do appear, however, to increase the incidence of endometrial cancer by about three to five times. Fortunately, this is a rare disease (incidence of about 1/100,000), and nearly all PME-associated endometrial cancers have been seen at early stages (perhaps because of an earlier presentation with estrogen-induced postmenopausal bleeding). Recently, some have advocated adding progestins to PME regimens to decrease the risk of endometrial cancer. However, the progestins may negate the beneficial effects of PME on serum lipids (estrogens raise HDL levels) and thus reduce the benefits of PME on coronary heart disease.

364. The answer is B. *(Wyngaarden, 19/e, pp 254–258.)* Contrary to common belief, systolic hypertension is as strong a risk factor for cardiovascular disease as is diastolic hypertension. Isolated systolic hypertension (ISH) is defined as a systolic pressure greater than 160 mmHg with a normal diastolic pressure (<90 mmHg). The prevalence of ISH increases with age in both men and women.

365. The answer is C. *(Wilson, 12/e, pp 1268–1281.)* Both types of inflammatory bowel disease are more common in whites than blacks and Asians. Jews have three to six times the incidence of non-Jews. There is no sex preference. The peak incidence of both diseases occurs between the ages of 15 and 35. There is an increased risk of colonic malignancy associated with ulcerative colitis, especially among those with pancolitis, who have a risk of cancer of about 40 percent after 24 years of the disease. However, prophylactic colectomy is no longer routine. Instead, periodic colonoscopy with biopsy of suspicious areas is recommended. Patients with pancolitis associated with Crohn's disease are at a slightly increased risk of colonic malignancy and should also have periodic colonoscopy.

366. The answer is C. *(Wilson, 12/e, p 967.)* Prognosis is related to the type and severity of coronary artery stenosis and the quality of the function of the left ventricle. Critical stenosis of the left main coronary artery, for example, is associated with a mortality of about 15 percent each year. The severity of myocardial ischemia (as reflected by angina or a markedly positive exercise test) is also predictive. Family history of heart disease is a risk factor for the incidence of coronary artery disease. Such a history, however, has not proved to be a predictor of prognosis for the disease. Elevated serum cholesterol levels, on the other hand, are associated with increased mortality following myocardial infarction. Treatment has been shown to be beneficial.

367. The answer is A. *(Last, Maxcy-Rosenau, 13/e, pp 389–391, 598, 627.)* Although most lead intake in humans is from ingestion of lead-contaminated food—about 0.1 mg of lead is ingested daily per person—the amount of lead that is absorbed after inhalation of lead-contaminated air is of greater significance because up to 50 percent of inhaled lead, compared with only as much as 10 percent of ingested lead, is absorbed and circulated by the blood. Because modern building codes usually require the replacement of lead domestic water-supply pipes by those made of copper or galvanized iron, drinking water has become a decreasing source of lead poisoning. The intake of lead through ingestion of lead-based paint is mainly a problem in children.

368. The answer is E. *(Last, Maxcy-Rosenau, 13/e, pp 551–558.)* Even though there is a great deal of literature on the adverse effects of workplace exposures, most of the nearly 10 million chemicals potentially used in U.S. workplaces have never been studied regarding their potential effects on human health. Animal data can only give approximations of human health risk, and these data are often unavailable or inapplicable. Recently, several U.S. regulatory agencies have issued testing guidelines for pharmaceuticals, food additives, pesticides, and household substances. Workplace exposures often have clinical findings similar to those of diseases caused by other factors; thus careful and complete medical histories are essential in diagnosing occupational disease. Unfortunately, most U.S. physicians are not trained to diagnose disease caused by occupational exposure, and this leads to an underdiagnosis of work-related diseases. There are some disincentives to investigating suspected cases of occupational disease, including a great deal of physician time and effort in getting exposure and toxicological data, the workers' compensation system, OSHA, and concern of physicians regarding jeopardizing the livelihoods of patients.

369. The answer is D. *(Last, Maxcy-Rosenau, 13/e, pp 535–538, 913–914.)* Once a back injury has been sustained, the muscles and ligaments of the injured areas are weaker than before the injury. Mechanical lifting devices should be used so that unassisted lifting can be avoided. Accident prevention programs should include consideration of a worker's physical condition and age as well as the frequency with which strenuous work is part of the work schedule. Unnatural or uncomfortable postures are often caused by improperly designed work stations. Work stations that are adjustable for individual workers can decrease musculoskeletal disorders.

370. The answer is A. *(Last, Maxcy-Rosenau, 13/e, pp 555, 587.)* More than 10 million chemicals are potentially used in U.S. workplaces, and PELs have not been established for most of these. PELs are different from the older occupational health standards, which were based on threshold limit values (TLVs). TLVs were calculated based on acute effects of maximum exposure only. Industrial hygienists can limit exposures by engineering controls, work-practice controls, and personal protective equipment. Employer-managed monitoring and sampling systems for toxic substances are now required by regulating agencies.

371. The answer is C. *(Last, Maxcy-Rosenau, 13/e, pp 947–958.)* When diagnosed according to the *DSM-III* criteria, rates of depression and anxiety disorders were found to be higher in 18 to 35 year olds and lower in older populations. The rate of alcoholism peaks in the early forties. In the U.S., Scandinavia, and England patients with schizophrenia are disproportionately likely to have been born during the winter or spring months. A two- to threefold increase in major depression in first-degree adult relatives of patients with depression has been reported. There is evidence that there is a genetic vulnerability to developing alcoholism. Males are much more likely to suffer from alcoholism than females, who have higher rates of depression and phobias than males. Before puberty males have more psychopathology than females, but this reverses itself during adolescence.

372. The answer is D. *(Behrman, 14/e, pp 490–492.)* Cocaine addiction among pregnant women has increased in recent times. These pregnancies may be complicated by premature labor and abruptio placentae. Withdrawal symptoms in the infant are unusual. Intrauterine growth retardation, microcephaly, intracranial hemorrhage, anomalies of the gastrointestinal and renal tracts, and developmental delay may be seen along with seizures in infants born to cocaine-addicted mothers. Facial abnormalities (including micrognathia), cardiac septal defects, minor joint and limb abnormalities, developmental delay, and mental deficiency are characteristic of fetal alcohol syndrome.

373. The answer is B. *(Behrman, 14/e, pp 131–132. Last, Maxcy-Rosenau, 13/e, p 996.)* Kwashiorkor results from a diet that is severely deficient in proteins and often sufficient or slightly deficient in calories. It occurs in toddlers after their weaning from breast milk to a diet high in carbohydrates and low in proteins and is characterized by changes in hair texture and color, ulcerated skin lesions, hepatomegaly, edema secondary to hypoalbuminemia, diarrhea, impaired liver function, and apathy.

374. The answer is D. *(Last, Maxcy-Rosenau, 13/e, p 728. USPS Task Force, pp 291, 293.)* Nicotine-containing chewing gum is a useful adjunct in helping smokers to quit. It is most successful in smokers who report high levels of addiction, but should be used in the context of a comprehensive program for cessation of smoking. Each stick of gum contains about 2 mg of nicotine, roughly the equivalent of one cigarette.

375. The answer is C. *(Last, Maxcy-Rosenau, 13/e, pp 142–144. USPS Task Force, pp 151–153.)* Mothers of infants with HSV infection are most often asymptomatic and HSV is unsuspected. There is no rapid, reliable, inexpensive method for screening for HSV yet. Because HSV-1 infection is relatively benign and most often latent, extensive measures for control of infection are not practical for the general population. However, immunocompromised persons and infants have an increased vulnerability, and it is appropriate to minimize their exposure to HSV. HSV transmission depends on direct contact with an HSV lesion or with secretions that contain the virus. Condoms protect more from disease transmitted by semen and vaginal secretions. Also, since many HSV infections are asymptomatic, condom use only during symptomatic periods does not completely prevent HSV transmission. HSV may be diagnosed visually or by viral culture, although the sensitivity of viral culture is highest during primary episodes and decreases with recurrent episodes. All hospital personnel with duties involving neonates or immunocompromised persons should be aware of the mode of transmission of HSV and take appropriate precautions.

376–379. The answers are 376-C, 377-E, 378-B, 379-A. *(Behrman, 14/e, pp 134–146.)* Scurvy due to *vitamin C deficiency* is characterized by pain and tenderness of the extremities, irritability, and hemorrhagic phenomena, all the result of defective formation of collagen. *Niacin deficiency* causes pellagra, which results in the four D's: disturbances of the gastrointestinal tract (*d*iarrhea), of the skin (*d*ermatitis), and of the nervous system (*d*elirium and *d*ementia). *Thiamine deficiency* leads to beriberi in which either myocardial disease (edema and cardiac failure) or neurologic signs predominate. *Vitamin A deficiency* leads to defects in epithelial cells of skin (hyperkeratosis) and to eye disorders (xerosis and keratomalacia, as well as night blindness). *Vitamin D deficiency* causes rickets in children and osteomalacia in adults; both conditions are due to the inadequate mineralization of bone.

380–384. The answers are 380-B, 381-B, 382-D, 383-A, 384-D. *(USPS Task Force, pp xlii–xlix. Hoekelman, pp 22–23.)* In the birth-to-18-month-old age group, leading causes of death include conditions originating in the perinatal period, congenital anomalies, infections, and nonmotor vehicle injuries (i.e., injuries not involving a motor vehicle). Routine blood testing is recommended in this age group as part of the neonatal screen, which may include screens for phenylketonuria, galactosemia, hypothyroidism, and hemoglobinopathies. (At all other ages, only high-risk patients should have blood tests performed.) Growth and development are monitored regularly. Counseling of parents should include nutrition, injury prevention, dental health, and effects of passive smoking. Routine immunization and chemoprophylaxis include ophthalmic antibiotics and diphtheria-pertussis-tetanus (DPT), measles-mumps-rubella (MMR), polio, *Haemophilus influenzae,* and hepatitis B vaccines.

In the 2-to-6-year-old age group leading causes of death are injuries (the majority do not involve motor vehicles), congenital anomalies, neoplasms, and homicide. Growth and development continues to be monitored and initial blood pressure measurements begin. Counseling includes exercise, dental hygiene, and diet with an emphasis on caloric balance. Dental visits begin. Injury prevention is again stressed and bicycle safety helmets recommended. Polio and DPT boosters are given at 4 to 6 years.

In the 7-to-12-year-old age group leading causes of death include injuries (the majority involve motor vehicles), neoplasms, congenital anomalies, and homicide. Growth, development, and blood pressure continue to be monitored. Diet, exercise, injury prevention, and dental health continue to be reviewed and appropriate patient and parent counseling performed. A measles booster is recommended at entry into either elementary or middle school.

In the 13-to-18-year-old age group leading causes of death include motor vehicle crashes, homicide, suicide, injuries not caused by motor vehicles, and cancer. Historical information is gathered and counseling given about diet, exercise, substance use, risk-taking behaviors, emotional well-being, and sexual practices. Given the importance of suicide in this age group, the history should include screening for stresses such as family difficulties, school problems, depression, and substance abuse. The physical examination should include cultures in sexually active adolescents. A tetanus-diphtheria booster (Td) is given at 14 to 16 years and every 10 years thereafter. Pertussis vaccination is not indicated in people over 7 years of age.

385–388. The answers are 385-B, 386-D, 387-C, 388-A. *(Benenson, 15/e, pp 50–52, 219–221, 418–420, 427–429, 450–451.) Necator americanus,* the American hookworm, enters the skin (usually of the foot) in the larval stage. The larvae are carried via lymphatics and blood to the lungs, where they migrate up the airways to be swallowed. They reach maturity and begin laying eggs in the intestine in 6 to 7 weeks. Autoinfection does not occur because the eggs are not infective for 7 to 10 days. Hookworm disease is primarily due to iron deficiency anemia from chronic gastrointestinal blood loss.

The life cycle of *Ascaris lumbricoides* begins when a person ingests infectious eggs. In the intestine these hatch into larvae, which migrate through the portal circulation to the lungs. After that, the life cycle is similar to that of *Necator americanus*: migration through the alveoli to airways, swallowing, and maturation and laying of eggs in the intestine. *Ascaris* eggs also are not immediately infectious; they require about 2 weeks of incubation. Thus ascariasis is also not directly transmissible from person to person.

The life cycle of *Strongyloides stercoralis* is similar to that of hookworm: larvae enter the skin, travel to the lungs, ascend the trachea, are swallowed, and develop into mature, egg-laying worms in the intestine. However, a crucial difference is that the eggs of *Strongyloides* may develop into infective filariform larvae even before leaving the host, and these larvae may pass through the perianal skin, lead to autoinfection, and increase the worm burden. This occurs most often in immunocompromised patients.

Taenia solium, the pork tapeworm, is acquired by ingestion of inadequately cooked pork that is infected with taenia cysticerci ("measly pork"). The cysticerci develop into egg-laying adult tapeworms in the intestine. However, unlike those of the beef tapeworm *(Taenia saginata),* eggs of *Taenia solium* are infective to humans. The ingested eggs develop into larvae, which then migrate throughout the soft tissues of the body, including the brain, eye, and heart.

Trichuris trichiura, or whipworm, has a relatively simple life cycle: after embryonated eggs are ingested, they develop into larvae, then adult worms. The worms lay eggs that are infectious for at least 3 weeks; thus, person-to-person transmission and autoinfection do not occur.

389–392. The answers are 389-C, 390-B, 391-E, 392-A. *(Benenson, 15/e, pp 255–257, 316–318, 364–366, 385–388, 474–477. Nelson, 10/e, p 41. Sanford, p 34.)* Sarcoptes scabiei is the name of the mite that causes scabies. The disease is due to the inflammatory response to the mite, which burrows under the skin and deposits eggs and feces. Treatment is with gamma benzene hexachloride (lindane; Kwell).

Pediculus humanus capitis, the head louse, causes epidemics among school children and institutionalized patients. A preparation of 1% permethrin (a synthetic pyrethrin) is the treatment of choice; lindane is a slightly less effective alternative.

Pediculus humanus corporis, the body louse, is the only louse that is an important vector of disease. It is the vector for epidemic typhus and relapsing fever, as well as for trench fever. It is most closely associated with severe poverty and lack of cleanliness.

Lyme disease is caused by a spirochete, *Borrelia burgdorferi,* transmitted to humans by infected ticks. The incubation period ranges from 3 days to a month after exposure. Treatment is with doxycycline in adults and amoxicillin and probenecid in children.

393–396. The answers are 393-E, 394-D, 395-A, 396-C. *(Behrman, 14/e, pp 110–112, 148.)* Fluorine is found in water, seafoods, and plant and animal foods depending upon the concentration of fluorine in the soil and water. It is retained when the intake is >0.6 mg/day and is excreted in urine and sweat. Supplementation for infants and children in areas without fluoridation of public water supplies is recommended.

Copper has many functions. It is a catalyst in hemoglobin formation, essential in production of red blood cells, and required for absorption of iron. The highest concentration is in the liver and central nervous system. It is excreted mainly via the intestinal wall and bile. Good dietary sources of copper are liver, oysters, meats, fish, and whole grains.

Zinc is a constituent of enzymes involved in carbon dioxide exchange and hydrolysis of protein. It is found in liver, bones, and red and white blood cells and is excreted mainly from the intestine. Children have a higher tissue concentration of zinc than adults.

Sodium helps to maintain cellular osmotic pressure, acid-base balance, and muscle and nerve function. It is absorbed easily from the intestine and excreted in the urine and sweat. It is coupled with chloride in many biochemical processes. Table salt, milk, eggs, seasonings, and preservatives are dietary sources of sodium.

Calcium is required for growth of bones and teeth, muscle contraction, nerve irritability, coagulation of blood, cardiac action, and production of milk. It is absorbed from the small intestine with the help of vitamin D. Most is excreted in the feces; the amount retained depends upon the growth rate. Good dietary sources include dairy products, green leafy vegetables, canned salmon, clams, and oysters.

397–401. The answers are 397-B, 398-A, 399-E, 400-B, 401-C. *(Wilson, 12/e, p 24.)* Screening programs for genetic diseases should be targeted at the ethnic or racial groups at highest risk. Blacks, for example, are at an increased risk of sickle cell disease. This includes both hemoglobin S and hemoglobin C. Blacks also have a higher incidence of other hemoglobinopathies, including both alpha and beta thalassemia. They also have a higher risk of glucose-6-phosphate dehydrogenase (G6PD) deficiency. G6PD deficiency is also seen in Chinese and Mediterranean people. Persons from the Mediterranean (including Greeks, Italians, and Sephardic Jews) are also at risk of familial Mediterranean fever and beta thalassemia. The Chinese are at increased risk of alpha thalassemia. Ashkenazic Jews (from Poland and Russia) are at increased risk of a variety of genetic diseases, including Tay-Sachs disease and Gaucher disease. Northern Europeans are at risk of cystic fibrosis. Alpha$_1$-antitrypsin deficiency is especially frequent in Scandinavians. Porphyria variegata is more common in whites from South Africa. Hemophilia is seen in all ethnic groups.

402–405. The answers are 402-B, 403-C, 404-D, 405-A. *(Benenson, 15/e, pp 1–7, 182–188, 417, 481–483. Last, Maxcy-Rosenau, 13/e, p 101.)* N. gonorrhoeae may cause urethritis, epididymitis, proctitis, cervicitis, and pelvic inflammatory disease, all of which may be associated with acute arthritis. Person-to-person transmission of G. lamblia, a cause of enteritis, is usually by feces of an infected person, especially in institutions and day-care centers. HPV can cause vulvar, vaginal, anal, and penile intraepithelial neoplasia, as well as carcinoma. HIV infection is associated with non-Hodgkin's lymphoma, Kaposi's sarcoma, *Pneumocystis carinii* pneumonia, cryptosporidiosis, toxoplasmosis, candidiasis, and other opportunistic infections. Group B streptococcus causes sepsis and meningitis in neonates and infants. The case fatality rate is 25 to 50 percent, and premature infants are at greatest risk for serious disease. The infection is acquired by person-to-person contact.

406–409. The answers are 406-E, 407-D, 408-B, 409-C. *(Benenson, 15/e, pp 1–7, 31–35, 430–433, 469–474.)* The principal means of controlling the AIDS epidemic is to effect reductions in high-risk behavior. Both antibody testing (to identify persons capable of transmitting the infection) and education (to inform people of which behaviors are most unsafe) are important components of such efforts. In addition, careful screening of donors, testing of the blood supply, and heat treatment of factor VIII concentrates have reduced transmission of the infection through blood products.

St. Louis encephalitis is caused by a virus in the flavivirus family, one of a group of *ar*thropod-*bo*rne ("arbo") viruses. The disease is transmitted by the bite of an infected mosquito. The viruses are difficult to culture; the diagnosis is generally suspected clinically and confirmed serologically. Control of the arboviral encephalitides requires control of the insect vector—in this instance elimination of breeding grounds for mosquitos, destruction of larvae, screening of sleeping and living quarters, and application of residual insecticides.

Unlike other species of salmonella, *Salmonella typhi,* the cause of typhoid fever, is found only in human beings; there is no animal reservoir. *S. typhi* is excreted in the feces of human carriers. Therefore, control of the disease primarily requires adequate sanitation. Sporadic cases continue to occur in the U.S.; these should be investigated by public health authorities, and the actual or probable source of the infection should be identified.

Immunization with tetanus toxoid is the best means of protection against tetanus. Since the causative organism is a normal inhabitant of the intestine of many animals (including human beings), the need for immunization will persist in spite of the present rarity of the disease. Persons who have sustained dirty wounds should receive tetanus immune globulin (TIG) unless they have an up-to-date status of tetanus vaccination (three past doses of tetanus toxoid, the most recent within the past 5 years).

410–413. The answers are 410-C, 411-A, 412-D, 413-B. *(Behrman, 14/e, pp 134–146.)* Vitamin C is necessary for normal collagen formation. Lack of vitamin C inhibits wound healing as well as causes scurvy. Numerous claims (each lacking substantiation) of benefits from vitamin E supplements have been made, including prevention of abortion, prevention of coronary heart disease, and improvement of lactation. One of the few demonstrated vitamin E deficiency states is a hemolytic anemia that occurs in premature babies. Rickets results from inadequate vitamin D intake that leads to failure of absorption of calcium and phosphate. Hemorrhagic disease of the newborn due to low levels of prothrombin and of other clotting factors can be prevented by administration of vitamin K_1 immediately after birth.

414–417. The answers are 414-B, 415-E, 416-D, 417-A. *(Benenson, 15/e, pp 318–322, 391–394, 420–426, 441–444.)* Infectious agents have developed a variety of means of transmission from one host to the next. Syphilis is spread by direct contact with exudates from early lesions of the skin or mucous membranes, or both of these, usually during sexual activity. Such lesions usually contain large numbers of spirochetes. Infection by direct contact with contaminated objects rarely occurs because of the lack of viability of the organisms outside the body.

During the diarrheal stage of shigellosis, large numbers of bacteria are excreted. The infectious dose for humans is as low as 100 bacteria; thus the disease is highly contagious, especially among young children who practice poor personal hygiene. Poor sanitation that allows contamination of food or water can cause large-scale outbreaks.

Pertussis, on the other hand, is transmitted in the respiratory secretions of infected persons during talking, coughing, sneezing, or singing. Direct person-to-person spread results from inhaling droplets that contain the bacteria. Children are most contagious during the initial (catarrhal) stage, during which large numbers of bacteria are present in the profuse and nasal secretions. The number of bacteria present in respiratory secretions falls rapidly during the second (paroxysmal) stage of the disease.

Trachoma, a chronic infection of the conjunctiva, is caused by *Chlamydia trachomatis* and is spread by contact with infected discharges from the eye. Direct person-to-person spread is the major means of transmission, although indirect mechanical transmission by flies may also occur. Trachoma is one of the major preventable causes of blindness in the world.

418–421. The answers are 418-D, 419-C, 420-E, 421-B. *(Benenson, 15/e, pp 142–144, 314–316, 427–429, 435–437. Last, Maxcy-Rosenau, 13/e, pp 268, 270, 274–275.)* Paragonimiasis is caused by the lung fluke, *Paragonimus westermani.* It has a complex life cycle in which larval stages undergo development in fresh-water crabs and other crustacea. Infection occurs by eating infected raw crabs. The disease, which affects the lungs and causes chronic cough and hemoptysis, occurs primarily in the Far East but has recently been reported in the western hemisphere.

Diphyllobothriasis is the disease caused by the fish tapeworm, *Diphyllobothrium latum,* which uses fresh-water fish as its intermediate host. One or two percent of infections are complicated by macrocytic anemia caused by interference with vitamin B_{12} absorption or by competition between the worm and the host for dietary vitamin B_{12}.

Toxocariasis is caused by the dog roundworm, *Toxocara canis.* The disease occurs mainly in children as the result of ingestion of soil contaminated with *Toxocara* eggs. Development of the *Toxocara* is incomplete in humans so that the larval stages migrate through the body— hence the term *visceral larva migrans.*

Cysticercosis is caused by the pork tapeworm, *Taenia solium.* Intestinal infection occurs by eating pork infested by cysts of *T. solium.* The adult tapeworm resides in the intestinal tract from which gravid proglottids (segments containing eggs) are shed in the feces. If the eggs hatch in the intestinal tract, the larvae can migrate throughout the body and often reach the brain. Cysticercosis is a common cause of epilepsy in Mexico and other developing countries.

422–425. The answers are 422-B, 423-C, 424-A, 425-B. *(Benenson, 15/e, pp 66–69, 72–74, 157–159, 324–329.)* The reservoir of *Candida albicans* is the human gastrointestinal tract. Candidal organisms, frequently part of the normal flora in the human body, cause disease only when host defenses are impaired as a result of disease, drug treatment, or altered immune response.

Numerous species of wild rodents are the natural reservoir of plague, in which transmission is through the bites of fleas infected with *Yersinia pestis.* While control of urban plague has been achieved in most of the world, plague still exists in rural areas of the United States, South America, Africa, and the Middle East, and in Central and Southeast

Asia. The potential of spread from the wild rodent reservoir to domestic rats, and then to humans, still exists.

Cattle, pigs, sheep, horses, reindeer, and goats are the main reservoirs of brucellosis. A systemic disease in humans, brucellosis may be acquired from raw milk or cheese from infected animals. It is also an occupational disease of farmers, abattoir workers, veterinarians, and others who have contact with animals that may be infected. Important economic losses can be caused by brucellosis in domestic animals.

Enterobiasis is an intestinal infection with the pinworm, *Enterobius vermicularis*. The most common symptom is anal itching, particularly at night. There is no animal reservoir, but infective eggs may survive in household dust for up to 2 weeks; hence careful daily sweeping or vacuuming for a few days after treatment may prevent reinfestation.

Provision of Health Services

DIRECTIONS: Each question below contains five suggested responses. Select the **one best** response to each question.

426. All the following statements about maternal and child health programs are true EXCEPT

(A) the first direct support for maternal and child health was the Shepard Towner Act in 1921

(B) Title V of the Social Security Act of 1935 provided for the federal government to assist in the support of crippled children's services

(C) funding for maternal and child health services decreased during the Reagan administration

(D) the maternal and child health block grants instituted by the Reagan administration decreased the autonomy of state and local government in the use of maternal and child health funds

(E) the proliferation of children's programs during the 60s and 70s created coordination problems as the result of the different agencies and organizations responsible for their administration

427. Which of the following health measures has the greatest potential for prevention of disease in the U.S.?

(A) Environmental modification
(B) Genetic counseling
(C) Immunization
(D) Modification of personal health behavior
(E) Screening tests

428. Which statement about Medicare is correct?

(A) Medicare is a federal and state cooperative program
(B) Medicare includes three parts: A, B, and C
(C) Part A of Medicare is financed by premiums from beneficiaries
(D) Part B of Medicare is reimbursed using the diagnosis-related groups (DRGs)
(E) None of the above

429. Guidelines for effective patient education and counseling include all the following EXCEPT

(A) obtaining commitment from patients to change behavior
(B) involving office staff
(C) involving patients in selection of risk factors that require change
(D) using a single strategy
(E) monitoring progress through follow-up contact

430. All the following statements about the resource-based relative value scale (RBRVS) are correct EXCEPT

(A) its purpose is to allow more equitable reimbursement of hospitals based on the cost of producing specific services
(B) it will lead to increasing reimbursement for primary care
(C) it will lead to decreased reimbursement for most surgery
(D) the proposed fees are similar to those already in place in Canada
(E) proponents hope that it will increase the incentive for physicians to spend more time with patients

431. Which of the following statements about long-term care is correct?

(A) There are more male than female patients in nursing homes
(B) Medicare generally covers the cost of nursing home care
(C) Home health services are the most costly component of long-term care
(D) There is a trend toward ownership of nursing homes by multihome, not-for-profit and for-profit entities
(E) None of the above

432. Principal findings of the United States Preventive Services (USPS) Task Force include all the following EXCEPT

(A) acute care visits are an appropriate setting for preventive services
(B) interventions that address personal health behavior are among the most effective
(C) more data and research are necessary to assess the effectiveness of various preventive services
(D) patients must assume greater responsibility for their own health
(E) screening tests should be applied uniformly

433. What proportion of total expenditures for health care in 1990 were covered by governmental programs?

(A) 22 percent
(B) 32 percent
(C) 42 percent
(D) 52 percent
(E) 62 percent

434. Which of the following statements regarding health maintenance organizations (HMOs) is correct?

(A) The number of HMOs and the number of subscribers to HMOs has declined over the last decade
(B) In a staff model HMO, the HMO contracts with a group
(C) HMOs have not been criticized for taking the healthiest patients and leaving ill patients to other health systems
(D) HMOs, like Blue Cross and Blue Shield, most often use "community rating" to set premiums
(E) None of the above

435. The largest proportion of the nation's hospital bill is covered by

(A) Medicare
(B) Medicaid
(C) private insurance
(D) other private payers
(E) out-of-pocket payments

436. Appropriate considerations for implementation of a screening test include all the following EXCEPT

(A) burden of suffering
(B) cost of screening test
(C) the physician's familiarity with the disease
(D) potential adverse effects of screening test
(E) efficacy of treatment

437. Physicians often fail to provide preventive medical services for all the following reasons EXCEPT

(A) insufficient financial reimbursement for preventive services
(B) insufficient time with patients during routine visits
(C) lack of published guidelines for routine care
(D) lack of routine visits by patients for health care maintenance
(E) uncertainty as to which services should be offered

438. Which of the following categories of service accounted for the largest proportion of health care costs in 1990?

(A) Hospitals
(B) Nursing homes
(C) Physicians
(D) Dentists
(E) Drugs

439. The proportion of Medicare's total expenditures used by the federal government to administer the program is

(A) 2 percent
(B) 4 percent
(C) 6 percent
(D) 8 percent
(E) 10 percent

440. All the following statements about the Employee Retirement Income and Security Act (ERISA) are true EXCEPT

(A) the Supreme Court has ruled states cannot regulate corporate self-funded health plans as the result of ERISA
(B) corporate self-funded health plans may avoid state-mandated required benefits in their plans
(C) small employers, who are not likely to be able to self-insure, are put at a disadvantage by these plans, as they must provide state-mandated benefits
(D) several states have challenged ERISA because of tax losses
(E) prenatal and well-baby care benefits are unaffected by ERISA

441. In *Healthy People: The Surgeon General's Report,* goals for lower death rates (fewer days of restricted activity for older adults) were set. By 1988 the goal was met for

(A) infants
(B) children
(C) adolescents
(D) adults
(E) older adults

442. Which of the following statements about international health is correct?

(A) Nearly 75 percent of the world's population live in the "developed" nations
(B) The World Health Organization (WHO) has established the goal of "health for all by the year 2000"
(C) The term *South* when used in discussions of international health includes most of the developed world
(D) Nongovernmental organizations played the major role in the eradication of smallpox
(E) None of the above

443. Which of the following statements about medical education and physician supply is correct?

(A) The Graduate Medical Education National Advisory Committee (GMENAC) reported that the supply of physicians would be in balance with needs by the year 2000

(B) The federal government continues to invest heavily in medical education in order to increase the supply of physicians

(C) The number of foreign medical graduates in the U.S. was minuscule prior to 1970, grew rapidly through the 1980s, and has tailed off somewhat

(D) The number of residency slots filled by foreign medical graduates continues to increase

(E) None of the above

444. All the following are among the "health promotion priority" areas in *Healthy People 2000* EXCEPT

(A) tobacco

(B) family planning

(C) occupational health and safety

(D) nutrition

(E) alcohol and other drugs

445. Which of the following statements about diagnosis-related groups (DRGs) is correct?

(A) The DRG is used to provide the reimbursement rates for Part B of Medicare

(B) The DRG payment is the same for urban and rural hospitals and is consistent across the U.S.

(C) There is a special payment pool for individuals who use far more than the expected volume of resources

(D) Manipulating the system by upgrading the DRG to get the highest possible reimbursement for an admission is called "churning"

(E) None of the above

446. In 1988, the highest infant mortality was reported for

(A) Canada

(B) East Germany

(C) Spain

(D) Singapore

(E) United States

447. Which of the following statements regarding use of health care services is correct?

(A) The use of services is lowest in young children
(B) Men in general use more health services than women
(C) While the difference has narrowed, African-Americans use more health services than whites
(D) Education seems to improve the likelihood that preventive services will be used
(E) None of the above

448. All the following are among Emerson's basic six functions for health departments EXCEPT

(A) vital statistics
(B) care for indigent patients
(C) maternal and child health
(D) health education
(E) environmental health

449. In analysis of cost-effectiveness, health benefits and costs that will not occur until some time in the future are often less highly valued. This process is called

(A) depreciation
(B) amortization
(C) discounting
(D) cost-shifting
(E) none of the above

450. Which of the following statements regarding for-profit health care in the U.S. is correct?

(A) Psychiatric hospitals and nursing homes are much more often operated for profit than are general hospitals
(B) For-profit hospitals generally have lower costs than non-profit hospitals
(C) After peaking in the late 1970s, the number of for-profit (proprietary) hospitals in the U.S. is decreasing
(D) Indicators of quality of hospital care, such as board certification of staff physicians and outcome of elective surgery, have generally shown that investor-owned chain hospitals are slightly superior to nonprofit or public hospitals
(E) None of the above

451. Which of the following categories of service accounted for the largest proportion of health care costs in the United States in 1984?

(A) Physicians
(B) Hospitals
(C) Drugs
(D) Nursing homes
(E) Dentists

452. An analysis of cost-effectiveness discloses that hemodialysis for a 50-year-old patient costs about $30,000 to $35,000 per quality-adjusted life year (QALY) saved. This indicates that

(A) hemodialysis is not cost-effective
(B) hemodialysis results in a relatively low quality of life
(C) placing a patient with renal failure on dialysis increases his or her life expectancy
(D) the annual incremental cost of hemodialysis is more than $40,000
(E) life expectancy of a patient on hemodialysis is less than 20 years

453. The number of Americans with no health insurance coverage is approximately

(A) 1,000,000
(B) 15,000,000
(C) 35,000,000
(D) 45,000,000
(E) 60,000,000

454. Which of the following statements about hospitals is correct?

(A) Nearly 40 percent of a hospital's beds are used by surgical patients
(B) The U.S. has an inadequate number of hospital beds
(C) Rural hospitals have been at an advantage with the advent of DRG reimbursement for Medicare services
(D) There has been a progressive decline in the number of hospitals affiliated with large hospital chains
(E) None of the above

455. Which of the following statements about Medicaid is correct?

(A) Medicaid is a federal program with national standards for eligibility
(B) Medicaid is available without concern for income to the elderly, permanently and totally disabled, and blind
(C) Among the mandated benefits, if the state is to receive Medicaid funding, are prescription drugs and ambulance service
(D) While recipients of Aid to Families with Dependent Children (AFDC) are the largest group of covered individuals, they consume less medical resources than other categories of Medicaid recipients
(E) None of the above

456. Which of the following statements about legal abortion in the U.S. is correct?

(A) The usual woman who has an abortion is nonwhite and older and has had previous children
(B) The majority of abortions occur outside the state of residence
(C) There is ample evidence of long-term psychological damage to a woman who has had an abortion
(D) There is evidence that an unmarried teenager who has an abortion is likely to complete school and have an improved economic status
(E) None of the above

457. Which of the following factors contributed to the increase in hospital costs over the past 10 years in the United States?

(A) Increased length of stay
(B) Increased competition among hospitals
(C) Increased numbers of hospital admissions
(D) Increased use of high-technology modes of diagnosis and treatment
(E) None of the above

458. Which of the following statements regarding group practice is correct?

(A) The first group practice was Roos-Loos in Los Angeles
(B) There continues to be a dramatic growth in the number of physicians who are in group practices
(C) Multispecialty group practices are the most common type of group practice in spite of the fact that they are smaller than single-specialty practices
(D) Most group practices contain more than 15 physicians
(E) None of the above

DIRECTIONS: Each group of questions below consists of lettered headings followed by a set of numbered items. For each numbered item select the **one** lettered heading with which it is **most** closely associated. Each lettered heading may be used **once, more than once, or not at all.**

Questions 459–462

Match each description below to the proper health care organization.

(A) Professional Review Organization (PRO)
(B) Health Maintenance Organization (HMO)
(C) Independent Practice Association
(D) Preferred Provider Organization (PPO)
(E) None of the above

459. Nonprofit association of physicians that reviews the quality of care provided to Medicare, Medicaid, and other patients

460. Group of providers who agree to provide services to specific groups of patients on a discounted fee-for-service basis

461. An organization that directly provides or arranges for all health services required by a defined population of prepaid clients

462. An organization that contracts with private physicians in the community to provide services to members of prepaid group health plans

Questions 463–466

For each function or program select the responsible agency.

(A) Food and Drug Administration
(B) Department of Agriculture
(C) Centers for Disease Control
(D) National Center for Health Statistics
(E) Environmental Protection Agency

463. Immunization and health education

464. Standards for drug manufacture

465. Guidelines of solid waste management

466. Women, Infants, and Children (WIC) food assistance program

Questions 467–470

Match each of the following.

(A) A private voluntary health agency
(B) A federal health agency
(C) A professional health organization
(D) An international health agency
(E) A health foundation

467. American Public Health Association

468. American Cancer Society

469. Pan American Health Organization

470. Centers for Disease Control

Provision of
Health Services
Answers

426. The answer is D. *(Last, Maxcy-Rosenau, 13/e, p 1095.)* While the absolute amount of funding for maternal and child health was cut during the Reagan administration, there was increased latitude in the use of the funds. They were allocated as block grants and state and local authorities had the discretion to use them for different maternal and child health needs. The Shepard Towner act was the first direct support from the federal government for maternal and child health. After being passed in 1921, it was repealed and then reincarnated with Title V of the Social Security Act, which also provided funding for crippled children's services. There was a proliferation of children's programs during the 60s and 70s. They were not well coordinated because various agencies of the federal government had responsibility for their administration.

427. The answer is D. *(USPS Task Force, pp xx–xxii.)* Although environmental modification, genetic counseling, immunization, and screening tests are important elements of preventive health, changing personal health behavior has the largest potential for improving public health in the United States, where the leading causes of death include heart disease, cancer, AIDS, injuries, and chronic obstructive pulmonary disease. Thus, alterations in personal health behaviors—such as smoking, diet, exercise, use of seatbelts, and safe sexual behavior—need to be stressed. Priorities would be different in developing countries where infectious disease and malnutrition are leading causes of death.

428. The answer is E. *(Last, Maxcy-Rosenau, 13/e, p 1077.)* Medicaid is a collaborative federal and state program. Medicare is a federal program with two parts: A and B. Part A covers mostly hospital-related expenses and Part B covers physician expenses. Part A is financed by an employee/employer tax, which is paid into a trust fund, while part B is financed partly through beneficiary premiums and partly from the U.S. general fund budget. Part A is reimbursed using DRGs, and Part

B is moving from "usual, customary, and prevailing reimbursement" to the resource-based relative value scale (RBRVS).

429. The answer is D. *(USPS Task Force, pp lix–lxi.)* One should use a combination of strategies in counseling patients for maximum effectiveness rather than rely on a single strategy. Individual counseling can be supplemented with classroom instruction, support groups, written material, and audiovisual aids. However, these materials are not a substitute for individual attention and feedback. Other principles for effective counseling in addition to those listed include counseling all patients, developing a therapeutic alliance with patients, ensuring that patients understand the relationship between health and behavior, working with patients to evaluate obstacles to behavior change, developing a behavioral modification program, involving office staff in promotion of behavioral change, and clinician role-modeling of health-promotion behaviors.

430. The answer is A. *(Wilson, 12/e, p 12.)* The RBRVS is a system for making *doctor's fees* more equitable—it does not address hospital reimbursement. It is meant to replace the "usual and customary rate" (UCR) schedule, which strongly rewarded technical procedures at the expense of cognitive services. For example, under the RBRVS the physician reimbursement for repair of an inguinal hernia would decrease from $503 to $233, and that for a coronary artery bypass (three grafts) from $3,652 to $1,936, while that for a limited office visit would increase from $19 all the way to $24. (That's equity?) Proponents hope that the scale will discourage overuse of procedures and encourage physicians to spend more time with patients.

431. The answer is D. *(Last, Maxcy-Rosenau, 13/e, p 1071.)* Residents of nursing homes are predominantly female and over 75 years of age and have multiple health problems. Medicaid, not Medicare, covers nursing home costs. Medicare will pay for a limited stay in a skilled nursing facility. Nursing homes usually are paid for "out-of-pocket" until the patient is indigent, and then Medicaid will pay. Nursing home care, not home health services, is the most expensive component of long-term care. While in the past nursing homes have tended to be small proprietary operations, there is a move toward larger, multihome systems, either nonprofit or proprietary.

432. The answer is E. *(USPS Task Force, pp xix–xxiii.)* The USPS Task Force was a 4-year, multidisciplinary, systematic effort to evaluate various preventive health measures. The task force published a book containing its assessment of 169 interventions in three different areas: screening, counseling, and immunization/chemoprophylaxis. The main finding was that personal health behavior (e.g., smoking, diet, exercise) is a major contributor to mortality and disability. The task force stressed the role of the physician as educator and counselor in addressing these behaviors while giving patients more responsibility for their own health. Other principal findings emphasized the need for greater *selectivity* in the application of screening tests, that is, careful consideration of the patient's age, sex, and other individual risk factors before applying screening tests. Evaluation of the screening tests revealed a need for better data to assess accurately the efficacy and appropriate frequency of the various measures. Additionally, since many patients only contact health care professionals for acute problems, the task force recommended including preventive health measures in illness visits for people with limited access to or inclination toward medical care.

433. The answer is C. *(Levit, Health Care Financing Rev 13:29, 1992.)* In 1990, 42 percent of health expenditures came from governmental programs. Out-of-pocket expenditures accounted for 20 percent, private health insurance covered 33 percent, and all other sources constituted 5 percent.

434. The answer is D. *(Williams, 4/e, pp 339–341.)* While the numbers of HMOs and their subscribers have not increased as rapidly as they did during the 70s and 80s, they continue to grow. In a group model HMO, the plan contracts with a group, as opposed to a staff model, where the physicians are on salary to the plan. HMOs have been criticized for "cream skimming," i.e., they take only healthy workers and leave sick people for others to care for. Under the provisions of the 1972 act that forced companies to offer HMO coverage if a federally qualified HMO was available, HMOs that wished to become federally qualified had to use community rating to set premiums, just as Blue Cross and Blue Shield do.

435. The answer is C. *(Levit, Health Care Financing Rev 13:52, 1992.)* Private insurance pays for 35 percent of the nation's total hospital bill. Medicare covers 27 percent and Medicaid 11 percent. Out-of-pocket payments account for 5 percent and other private insurance covers 5.5 percent, with the remainder provided from a variety of sources.

436. The answer is C. *(USPS Task Force, pp xxvii–xxxiii.)* A variety of factors need to be considered before instituting any preventive health measure, including a screening test. The burden of suffering includes both the severity and the prevalence of the disease. Other things being equal, rare diseases are less important than more common diseases, and illnesses of minor clinical significance less important than illnesses with high morbidity and mortality. Recall also that the positive predictive value of a screening test increases as prevalence of the disease increases. Another requirement for the rational institution of a screening program is the availability (both technically and socioeconomically) of effective treatment. If no effective intervention is available for a disease, screening will only serve to produce a lead-time bias: an apparent prolongation of life by detecting a disease at an earlier stage without a true impact on survival. Additional criteria for screening tests include cost, efficacy, and potential adverse effects. The ideal screening test is inexpensive and reliable (high sensitivity and specificity). Low specificity and prevalence lead to many patients with false positive results, who must then undergo further evaluation and therapy with the attendant risk of iatrogenic morbidity. The targeting of screening tests to populations specifically at risk rather than to the population as a whole will limit costs, reduce the number of false positives, and hence decrease the adverse effects of screening.

A physician's familiarity with a disease is not an important consideration when compared with the above criteria. Primary care physicians can screen for quite uncommon diseases with which they are unfamiliar (e.g., galactosemia) as long as they know where to refer patients who test positive. As medical science progresses, screening tests offer a means of educating both practitioner and patient.

437. The answer is C. *(USPS Task Force, pp xx–xxi.)* A variety of factors enter into an overall lack of preventive medical services. Many Americans are uninsured or underinsured, have no regular medical provider, and seek care only in urgent situations. These people do not have routine visits for health care maintenance. For these people the acute care visit is an important setting for the delivery of preventive health services because it may be their only contact with health care professionals. Furthermore, preventive services are poorly reimbursed compared with more invasive services. This financial disincentive, combined with time pressures during routine visits, discourages physicians from providing preventive measures such as investigation of behavioral risk factors and counseling. Paradoxically, more invasive and financially rewarding measures may be encouraged, such as treadmill testing, which, while appropriate to high-risk populations, should not be applied to the general population.

Physicians interested in preventive health measures may be uncertain as to which measures to institute. There is no lack of published guidelines for preventive health; recommendations are available from a variety of sources including professional and volunteer organizations as well as scientific and governmental bodies. Other sources of physician uncertainty may include skepticism of the efficacy of preventive measures and concerns of subjecting an asymptomatic, healthy person to possibly harmful interventions.

438. The answer is A. *(Levit, Health Care Financing Rev 13:29, 1992.)* Hospital costs accounted for 38 percent of national health expenditures in the U.S. in 1990, twice as much as the cost of physician services (19 percent). The proportions of costs devoted to nursing homes, drugs, and dentists were 8, 7, and 7 percent, respectively.

439. The answer is A. *(Levit, Health Care Financing Rev 13:36–37, 1992.)* In 1990, private health insurance firms had an administrative cost of 14.2 percent and Medicare was 2 percent. A major reason has to do with the nature of Medicare as an entitlement: there is an eligibility determination only once; a sales force does not have to be paid; the premiums are not, with the exception of a small portion of part B, collected; and there are no shareholders who must receive return on equity.

440. The answer is E. *(Williams, 4/e, pp 347–348.)* ERISA was passed in 1974 and the Supreme Court ruled in 1985 that self-insured companies were exempt from state regulation, including the items that should be provided in a benefit package. Such regulations were frequently mandated by states to assure that certain important benefits, like prenatal and well-baby care, were covered by plans doing business in the state. This has worked to the disadvantage of small businesses that are not able to self-insure because of their small size and as a result must provide the state-mandated benefits while a larger employer does not. A number of states have attacked ERISA exclusions, without success so far, because of lost tax revenue.

441. The answer is B. *(USDHHS, p 4.)* The goals and their status as of 1988 were as follows:

Age Group	1990 Goal	1988 Status
Infants	35% lower death rate	28% lower
Children	20% lower death rate	21% lower
Adolescents	20% lower death rate	13% lower
Adults	25% lower death rate	21% lower
Older Adults	20% fewer days of restricted activity	17% fewer

442. The answer is B. *(Last, Maxcy-Rosenau, 13/e, pp 1129–1130.)* Seventy-five percent of the world's population live in developing nations, which contain only 20 percent of the world's wealth. The WHO has established the goal (and slogan) of "health for all by the year 2000." *North* according to the Brandt Commission refers to the developed nations, while *South* includes the developing world, such as Africa and Latin America. The WHO played the major role in the worldwide eradication of smallpox. It was WHO that established and supported the Commission on the Worldwide Eradication of Smallpox.

443. The answer is C. *(Williams, 4/e, pp 271–273.)* The GMENAC thought the U.S. would have a surplus of 70,000 physicians in 1990 and 145,000 in the year 2000. After the release of the GMENAC report there was a steady decline in the funds available in the Health Professions Assistance Act to support medical education because the U.S. was producing too many physicians. Due to preferential visa treatment, there was a steady increase in the total number of foreign medical graduates through the early 70s, along with a progressively increasing number in residency slots in the U.S. With changes in those preferential immigration laws and efforts to decrease the number of foreign medical graduates in residency slots, there has been a progressive decline in the numbers of foreign medical graduates.

444. The answer is C. *(USDHHS, p 7.)* "Health promotion priority" areas include physical activity and fitness, nutrition, tobacco, alcohol and other drugs, family planning, mental health, violent and abusive behavior, and community-based programs. Occupational health and safety are included in the "health protection priority" areas, along with unintentional injuries, environmental health, food and drug safety, and oral health.

445. The answer is C. *(Williams 4/e, pp 320–324.)* The DRG is used to calculate the reimbursement rate for part A of Medicare. The DRGs are adjusted annually for urban/rural differences and by region of the country. If patients exceed a certain cost or length of stay, they become an "outlier" and are eligible for extra payments to cover a portion of the cost beyond the limit. Upgrading the DRG to obtain a higher reimbursement is called "DRG creep"; "churning" is readmitting the patient several times for related procedures or diagnosis, which results in additional DRG payments.

446. The answer is E. *(Last, Maxcy-Rosenau, 13/e, pp 1133–1135.)* In 1987 the United States tied with Italy for 21st place worldwide in infant mortality, with 10.1 deaths per 1000 live births. Japan ranked first (5.0) with provisional rates for 1988 even lower. Other countries ranking above the United States include Canada (7.3), Singapore (7.4), East Germany (8.5), and Spain (8.5). These comparisons also hold true if one only considers infant mortality for whites in the United States (8.6). Advocates for stronger prenatal care use these data to illustrate the inadequacies of the delivery system for health care in the United States.

447. The answer is D. *(Williams, 4/e, pp 60–61.)* The age curve for use of services is curvilinear, with older persons and young children likely to have higher use than those in the middle. Women tend to use more services than men; whites appear to use more services than African-Americans. Better-educated people are more likely to be immunized, seek physicians earlier in pregnancy, have screening tests done, and see their physician for a preventive examination.

448. The answer is B. *(Williams, 4/e, p 85.)* Emerson's basic six functions of a health department are vital statistics, maternal and child health, health education, laboratory, environment, and control of communicable diseases. There continues to be controversy about the role of the health department in providing personal health services to the indigent.

449. The answer is C. *(Wilson, 12/e, p 13.)* *Discounting* is the term used to describe the reduced value of costs and benefits first realized in the future. It is dependent on monetary inflation, as well as on the extent to which society wishes to invest today's dollars for future health. Depreciation and amortization refer to the process by which capital investments are written off over a period of years. Cost-shifting occurs when the costs of care for some people (usually poor and uninsured) are shifted to others who are able to pay the bills.

450. The answer is A. *(Gray, N Engl J Med 314:1523–1528, 1986. Relman, N Engl J Med 303:963–970, 1980.)* For-profit health care in the U.S. has been increasing dramatically and has expanded from nursing homes and psychiatric hospitals, which traditionally have been more frequently proprietary, to general hospitals. Clinical laboratories, home care, and hemodialysis centers are also substantially for-profit industries. For-profit hospitals do not generally have lower costs than nonprofit hospitals, but collections per case from third party payers have been 15 to 20 percent higher in for-profit hospitals. Indicators of quality of care have not shown much difference between investor-owned hospital chains and nonprofit hospitals, although historical problems with proprietary nursing homes suggest that continued caution is indicated regarding quality of care in for-profit hospitals.

451. The answer is B. *(Levit, Health Care Financing Rev 13:29, 1992. Office of National Cost Estimates, Health Care Financing Rev 11:1–41, 1990.)* Hospital costs accounted for 38 percent of national health expenditures in the United States in 1988, twice as much as costs of physician services (19 percent). Nursing homes accounted for 8 percent.

452. The answer is C. *(Wilson, 12/e, pp 5–11.)* Hemodialysis must increase life expectancy, otherwise it would result in a situation in which there is cost per year of life lost. Quality-adjusted life years (QALYs) are an attempt to compare the value of life in the presence of a chronic medical problem (like the need for hemodialysis) with perfect health, which is assigned a value of 1.0; the quality adjustment for patients on hemodialysis would differ among patients, but would be less than 1.0—perhaps, say, 0.9. In its most simple formulation, cost per QALY saved is simply cost divided by the quality adjustment. Thus cost is cost-effectiveness times the quality adjustment, and the cost of hemodialysis (since the quality adjustment is less than 1.0) must be less than $30,000 to $35,000 per year. There is no way to determine life expectancy or quality of life in this situation, nor can one ever say whether a technology is cost-effective unless one asks against what its cost-effectiveness is to be compared.

453. The answer is C. *(Last, Maxcy-Rosenau, 13/e, pp 1076–1077.)* Approximately 37,000,000 Americans have no health insurance at all. Tens of millions more are underinsured, often with hefty deductibles and copayments or coverage only for inpatient acute services. Even those who have insurance face losing it if they change their employment.

454. The answer is A. *(Last, Maxcy-Rosenau, 13/e, pp 1066–1068.)* As the result of Hill-Burton legislation and changing reimbursement patterns, there has been a tremendous decline in hospital occupancy; thus, the U.S. has too many hospital beds. Rural hospitals have suffered as the result of the DRG method of payment, and a disproportionate number of the hospitals that have closed as the result of DRGs have been rural. Finally, there has been an increase in the number of hospitals affiliating with chains, not only proprietary but also not-for-profit hospitals.

455. The answer is D. *(Williams, 4/e, pp 312–313.)* Medicaid is a federal/state program and financial eligibility is determined on a state-by-state basis. To receive Medicaid benefits you must be poor, as defined by the state, *and* be blind, aged, permanently and totally disabled, or a recipient of Aid to Families with Dependent Children. The mandated benefits do not include prescription drugs or ambulance service. While there are fewer aged and permanently and totally disabled recipients than those who receive AFDC, the former two categories use the most health resources because AFDC recipients are younger and healthier.

456. The answer is D. *(Last, Maxcy-Rosenau, pp 1107–1108.)* The usual abortion patient is unmarried, white, and under 25 years old and has had no previous pregnancy. Most abortions are performed in the state of residency. There is not enough evidence, pro or con, for the Surgeon General to issue a report on the psychological sequelae of abortion. Studies do demonstrate that teenage African-American women who have abortions are more likely to finish high school and have a better economic status 5 years later.

457. The answer is D. *(Williams, 4/e, pp 159–162.)* Over the past 10 years there has been increasing use of x-rays, laboratory tests, and high-technology therapy. The increase in costs has occurred despite a leveling off of hospital admissions and shorter hospital stays. Some of the increase, ironically, is due to the cost of complying with regulations whose goal was containment of costs.

458. The answer is B. *(Williams, 4/e, pp 120–121.)* The first group practice was the Mayo Clinic in Rochester, Minnesota. There continues to be a dramatic growth in the number of group practices, but particularly in the number of physicians who choose group practice. The most common type of group is the single-specialty group. There are fewer multispecialty groups, but they tend to be larger than single-specialty groups. The average number of physicians in a group is 9, and the majority of physicians tend to practice in groups with less than 15 physicians.

459–462. The answers are 459-A, 460-D, 461-B, 462-C. *(Williams, 4/e, pp 325–326, 339–341, 363, 392–393.)* Review of the quality of care is the purview of Professional Review Organizations (PROs), formerly called Professional Standards Review Organizations, which were established in the 1972 Social Security Amendments. PROs may contract with businesses as well as with the Department of Health and Human Services (DHHS) to monitor quality of care and hospital utilization.

Preferred Provider Organizations (PPOs) are groups of providers that make special arrangements with insurers to provide services to their customers on a discounted basis, i.e., to accept lower levels of reimbursement than their usual rates. An example is the Blue Cross "Prudent Buyer Plan," in which patients who are willing to obtain care from preferred providers can save on coinsurance and deductibles.

Health Maintenance Organizations (HMOs) provide comprehensive health care services on a prepaid basis. First developed around the turn of the century, they were bitterly opposed by organized medicine. In the early 1970s, legislation encouraging their development was passed, which led to the establishment of 166 HMOs by 1975 and to 323 HMOs covering 15 million members by 1985.

Independent Practice Associations (IPAs) are a more recent development. Whereas HMOs have traditionally served their patients by employing full-time physicians in their own clinics and medical centers, IPAs allow private physicians to contract with HMOs to provide services to enrolled patients.

463–466. The answers are 463-C, 464-A, 465-E, 466-B. *(Green, 6/e, pp 120, 441–442, 444, 455–459.)* The Centers for Disease Control's responsibilities are to provide surveillance and investigation of epidemic diseases, to promote disease-control programs, to provide expert laboratory assistance to state and local health departments, and to promote immunization and health education programs.

The Food and Drug Administration (FDA) was established in 1906 to enforce the laws that regulated interstate transport and quality of drugs and food. The FDA, which received its current name in 1931, assures that safe and effective prescription drugs are sold to the public. To do this, the FDA tests products, sets standards for production and quality control, and judges claims of safety and efficacy.

The Environmental Protection Agency (EPA) is responsible for protection and promotion of environmental quality. The EPA sets guidelines for solid waste disposal, for hazardous waste control, for recovery of resources from wastes, and for the screening of potentially hazardous chemicals prior to production and distribution.

The Women, Infants, and Children (WIC) food assistance program is the largest federally funded state health program. It is administered by the U.S. Department of Agriculture and provides supplemental food for pregnant and nursing women, infants, and children.

467–470. The answers are 467-C, 468-A, 469-D, 470-B. *(Green, 6/e, pp 456–459, 465, 470–471, 528.)* Professional health organizations are groups formed by persons who have met prescribed standards of training and certification and whose purposes are to promote the interests of the profession and to serve the public. An example is the American Public Health Association, founded in 1872, which establishes standards and guidelines related to public health; implements public health education through its journal, other publications, and meetings; and provides expert testimony to legislative groups.

The American Cancer Society, founded in 1913, is an example of a nonprofit, voluntary health agency, which was organized to disseminate knowledge about cancer and is supported by voluntary donations.

The Pan American Health Organization, established in 1901, is an international health agency representing the nations of the Americas. Its major concern has been control of communicable diseases. It has been integrated into the World Health Organization and serves as the regional office for the Americas.

The Centers for Disease Control, formerly known as the Communicable Disease Center, is a branch of the United States Public Health Service. It is the federal agency responsible for surveillance of communicable diseases in the United States.

Legal and Ethical Issues

DIRECTIONS: Each question below contains five suggested responses. Select the **one best** response to each question.

471. Which of the following statements about child abuse is correct?

(A) Child abusers are most often unrelated to the child
(B) Most child abusers have psychotic or antisocial personalities
(C) The most common sites for bruises associated with abuse are over the forehead, anterior tibia, and other bony prominences
(D) It is unnecessary to report child abuse in some jurisdictions
(E) None of the above

472. Which of the following statements regarding domestic battering of women is correct?

(A) Most instances of spouse abuse occur as isolated incidents
(B) Among married women, less than 2 percent are beaten by their husbands over the course of a year
(C) The majority of instances of woman battering are caused by alcohol abuse
(D) Presenting complaints among abused women seeking medical attention are often nonspecific
(E) None of the above

473. In keeping with the principles for providing occupational medical services, physicians should do all the following EXCEPT

(A) practice on a scientific basis with objectivity and integrity
(B) actively oppose and strive to correct unethical conduct in relation to occupational health science
(C) seek consultation concerning the individual or the workplace wherever indicated
(D) release medical information to the employers whenever requested by the employer
(E) avoid allowing medical judgment to be influenced by any conflict of interest

474. All the following diseases require notification of public health authorities in the U.S. EXCEPT

(A) aseptic meningitis
(B) hepatitis
(C) mumps
(D) campylobacteriosis
(E) cholera

475. Which of the following statements regarding informed consent for medical treatment is correct?

(A) Physicians must disclose risks of a specific treatment, but are not required to discuss alternative treatments if they are less effective
(B) Because risks of procedures may be frightening, it is best to defer the discussion until after the patient has been sedated
(C) In order to be valid, informed consent must be written and include the patient's signature and the date
(D) The primary factor in the physician's responsibility to inform the patient of an adverse effect is the frequency of that effect
(E) None of the above

476. Cholera and plague are reportable diseases according to the 1969 International Health Regulations. Other reportable diseases include all the following EXCEPT

(A) hepatitis B
(B) malaria
(C) paralytic poliomyelitis
(D) yellow fever
(E) smallpox

477. The carelessness or dereliction of duty by a professional person is called

(A) criminal negligence
(B) malfeasance
(C) misfeasance
(D) malpractice
(E) none of the above

478. In order for a patient to recover damages due to negligence, each of the following elements must be present EXCEPT

(A) duty to care
(B) breach of duty
(C) injury
(D) nonfeasance
(E) proximate cause

479. All the following statements about "Good Samaritan" laws are true EXCEPT

(A) they have been enacted by most states
(B) they are designed to encourage health professionals to provide assistance in emergency situations
(C) they free providers from liability for gross or criminal negligence
(D) they generally require that assistance be rendered without payment or expectation of payment for services
(E) they may apply to both professionals and laypersons

480. When debating whether providing or withholding medical treatment is ethical, the LEAST important consideration of those listed below is

(A) indications for medical intervention
(B) expected quality of life
(C) patient's preferences
(D) physician's preferences
(E) economic factors

481. As organ transplantation has become more common, guidelines have been developed to govern organ donation. The Uniform Anatomical Gift Act does all the following EXCEPT

(A) allow partial donation
(B) free health care personnel from civil and criminal liability when acting in good faith
(C) limit which physicians may certify time of death
(D) provide for revocation of a donation
(E) require express, documented consent by the donor

482. Which of the following patients is incompetent and should receive medical care against his or her expressed wishes?

(A) A 32-year-old Jehovah's Witness who had refused transfusions for a ruptured ectopic pregnancy and is now unresponsive postoperatively with a hematocrit of 8 percent

(B) An anxious, frightened 48-year-old patient who refuses surgery for gastric cancer because "it's too scary"

(C) A 55-year-old executive with chest pain and ECG changes who refuses hospitalization because of "an important business deal"

(D) An active 83-year-old diabetic who refuses treatment for a gangrenous foot ulcer because "I'm going to die anyway"

(E) None of the above

483. Physicians have obligations to report all the following EXCEPT

(A) accidental gunshot wounds
(B) births and deaths
(C) certain communicable diseases
(D) child abuse
(E) substance abuse

484. All the following statements are true EXCEPT

(A) the Hippocratic Oath contains such ethical precepts as beneficence, confidentiality, and nonmaleficence

(B) both Socrates and Plato produced a treatise specifically devoted to the ethics of medicine

(C) among the prima facie ethical principles developed during the 1960s and 1970s are justice, autonomy, and beneficence

(D) the ethics of caring suggest that women are more caring than men in the way they approach ethical decisions

(E) clinical bioethics focus on the clinical realities of moral choices on a day-to-day basis

485. The Hippocratic Oath specifically includes all the following elements EXCEPT

(A) respect for and commitment to teachers
(B) proscriptions against abortion
(C) proscriptions against euthanasia
(D) proscriptions against sexual misconduct
(E) proscriptions against substance abuse

486. All the following principles are among the Department of Health and Human Services (DHHS) guidelines for ethical research EXCEPT

(A) confidentiality is adequately protected
(B) informed consent is obtained if appropriate
(C) subjects are adequately compensated for time or pain
(D) data are monitored to ensure safety of subjects
(E) additional safeguards are instituted for vulnerable patients

487. A physician fills out a death certificate as follows:
*Immediate cause of death—*pulmonary embolism
*Due to—*deep venous thrombosis
*Due to—*pancreatic cancer
She notes that a liver biopsy was performed prior to death. In the U.S. vital statistics, this death would be recorded as due to

(A) pulmonary embolism
(B) deep venous thrombosis
(C) pancreatic cancer
(D) Trousseau's syndrome
(E) complication of liver biopsy

488. One of your patients who has metastatic breast cancer develops shortness of breath. She presents to the emergency department, where you diagnose pericarditis, which is confirmed by echocardiography. Soon after, cardiac tamponade occurs and she develops ventricular tachycardia and then ventricular fibrillation. Cardiopulmonary resuscitation is unsuccessful. Despite your request, her family refuses an autopsy. How should you indicate the cause of death on the death certificate for this woman?

(A) Cardiopulmonary arrest due to ventricular fibrillation due to ventricular tachycardia
(B) Ventricular fibrillation due to cardiac tamponade due to pericarditis
(C) Pericarditis
(D) Breast cancer
(E) The death certificate should not be filled out; this is a coroner's case

DIRECTIONS: Each group of questions below consists of lettered headings followed by a set of numbered items. For each numbered item select the **one** lettered heading with which it is **most** closely associated. Each lettered heading may be used **once, more than once, or not at all.**

Questions 489–491

Match each of the following legal cases with the relevant subject matter.

(A) Abortion
(B) Duty to warn
(C) Informed consent
(D) Malpractice liability
(E) Termination of life support

489. *Darling v. Charleston Community Memorial Hospital*

490. *In re Quinlan*

491. *Tarasoff v. Regents of the University of California*

Questions 492–494

Match the following situations with the appropriate legal claim.

(A) Abandonment
(B) Assault
(C) Battery
(D) False imprisonment
(E) Misdiagnosis

492. Informed consent is not obtained for a surgical procedure

493. A physician does not follow up after the acute stage of an illness

494. Restraints are used on a competent, nonviolent patient

Questions 495–497

Match the following actions to the underlying ethical principle.

(A) Autonomy
(B) Beneficence
(C) Euthanasia
(D) Supererogation
(E) Utilitarianism

495. A state legislature decides to allocate funds to prenatal care instead of intensive care nurseries

496. A person with AIDS refuses intubation for *Pneumocystis carinii* pneumonia and dies

497. A 27-year-old woman donates a kidney to her 17-year-old brother who has end-stage renal disease

DIRECTIONS: The group of questions below consists of four lettered headings followed by a set of numbered items. For each numbered item select

A	if the item is associated with	(A) **only**
B	if the item is associated with	(B) **only**
C	if the item is associated with	**both** (A) and (B)
D	if the item is associated with	**neither** (A) nor (B)

Each lettered heading may be used **once, more than once, or not at all.**

Questions 498–500

(A) Claims-made policy for professional liability insurance
(B) Occurrence policy for professional liability insurance
(C) Both
(D) Neither

498. Events that occurred prior to institution of the policy are covered

499. Amount payable is limited

500. Notification of occurrence and claim is required

Legal and
Ethical Issues
Answers

471. The answer is C. *(Behrman, 14/e, pp 78–83.)* The abuser is a related caregiver or male friend of the mother in 95 percent of cases. Over 90 percent of abusing parents have neither psychotic nor criminal personalities. They tend to be lonely, unhappy, angry adults under heavy stress. It is necessary to report child abuse in all U.S. jurisdictions immediately.

472. The answer is D. *(Last, Maxcy-Rosenau, 13/e, pp 1040–1044.)* In three surveys, the frequency of spouse abuse was 3.8 percent (in a national study), 8.5 percent (in Texas), and 10 percent (a Harris poll in Kentucky). Spouse abuse most often occurs in an ongoing pattern. Although patients may present with specific injuries, often complaints are related to injuries incurred in the past and are not recognized by medical personnel as related to spouse abuse. Although alcohol abuse is associated with domestic violence, it seems to be more often the excuse than the cause.

473. The answer is D. *(Last, Maxcy-Rosenau, 13/e, p 1194.)* The code for physicians who provide occupational medical services specifically bars providing information to an employer, except in certain circumstances. The code states that physicians should "treat as confidential whatever is learned about the individuals served, releasing information only when required by law or by over-riding public health considerations, or to other physicians at the request of the individual according to traditional medical ethical practice; and should recognize that employers are entitled to counsel about the medical fitness of individuals in relation to work, but are not entitled to diagnoses or details of a specific nature."

474. The answer is D. *(Last, Human Ecology, pp 103–130.)* All of the diseases listed, though they may be of low frequency (e.g., cholera), are notifiable diseases in the U.S. except campylobacteriosis. If there were an acute outbreak of common-source *Campylobacter* gastroenteritis that would also be reportable, as all epidemics are notifiable diseases.

475. The answer is E. *(Hoekelman, pp 35–38.)* To make an informed decision regarding treatment, patients need to be informed not only of the risks of the treatment, but also of its expected efficacy, and the expected efficacy and risks of alternative treatments. Consent should be obtained before sedation, not only because the discussion should take place while the patient is lucid, but also because sedation itself may be associated with risks. Consent may be obtained verbally. As a general rule, the need to inform patients of adverse effects of treatment is more dependent on the severity of the adverse effect than on its frequency.

476. The answer is A. *(Benenson, 15/e, pp xxiv–xxv.)* The selection of infectious diseases to be reported is usually a matter of local discretion. The reporting of cholera, plague, smallpox, yellow fever, paralytic poliomyelitis, and malaria (as well as viral influenza, louse-borne typhus fever, and louse-borne relapsing fever) is universally required in all countries subject to the 1969 International Health Regulations or agreements at the 22nd World Health Assembly. Because of their potential for causing epidemics, cases of these diseases should be immediately reported to local health authorities.

477. The answer is D. *(Pozgar, 4/e, p 16.)* Legally, negligence is defined in terms of the expected behavior of a "reasonably prudent person" in a certain situation. Criminal negligence is the reckless disregard for the well-being of another and would usually constitute gross negligence as opposed to ordinary negligence. Malpractice is the negligence of a professional person such as a physician, nurse, or lawyer. Malfeasance is the performance of an unlawful act. Misfeasance is the improper performance of a lawful act that results in injury to another.

478. The answer is D. *(Pozgar, 4/e, pp 17–23.)* Duty to use due care is the legal obligation of one party to protect another party by conforming to a specific standard of care. This duty arises from the doctor-patient, nurse-patient, or hospital-patient relationship and can be created by a telephone call or by displaying an emergency room sign. A physician passing an accident victim on the highway has a moral obligation to stop and render assistance, but there is no legal obligation because the doctor-patient relationship is not established.

Breach of duty is the failure to fulfill this duty according to the prevailing standard of care. Standard of care is based on the behavior of a hypothetical "reasonably prudent person" with similar training and knowledge. This standard may be a national or an "industry" standard as opposed to a community standard. Expert witness testimony is often used in attempts to define this standard.

Unless injuries actually occur, damages cannot be awarded. Malpractice may have been committed, but if there were no untoward results, damages due to negligence cannot be recovered. The legal term *injuries* includes mental anguish and violation of rights and privileges in addition to physical harm.

Finally, causation must be established. This must be a reasonable and close relationship, but it need not be direct. For example, an accident victim who has never encountered the physician may receive damages for physician negligence when injured by a patient who is driving under the influence of a drug prescribed by the physician if the patient received no warnings concerning the drug's intoxicating nature.

Nonfeasance is a negligent act of omission, failing to perform an act that a reasonably prudent person would be expected to perform under the same circumstances. This would satisfy the criteria for breach of duty, but in itself is not necessary for the awarding of damages.

479. The answer is C. *(Pozgar, 4/e, pp 261–262.)* Good Samaritan laws free health professionals from ordinary negligence in emergency situations where no preexisting duty to use due care exists. They do not apply to acute situations in the emergency room, but rather are designed to encourage health professionals to volunteer their assistance in emergency situations by eliminating liability concerns. No expectation of financial compensation can exist, for this implies a professional/contractual relationship. Good Samaritan laws have been enacted by almost all states, but statutes vary; they may apply to laypersons as well. While the laws free providers from liability for ordinary negligence, they do not free persons from liability for gross or criminal negligence or for "willful or wanton" misconduct.

480. The answer is D. *(Jonsen, 2/e, pp 4–8, 92–94.)* The overriding consideration in questions of clinical ethics is the patient's preference, which reflects the principle of autonomy. In most cases physicians are morally obligated to respect the patient's wishes, and strong efforts to identify the patient's preferences need to be made. Another important general category for consideration is the indication for medical intervention. Physicians need to make objective, educated judgments about the risks and benefits of diagnostic and therapeutic efforts. Measures that clearly are not medically indicated need not be pursued, even in the face of a patient's preference. Examples here include "Do Not Resuscitate" (DNR) orders and termination of ineffective therapy in terminally ill patients. Considerations of quality of life include elements of the patient's preference, disease progression, and efficacy of treatment. If the patient's preferences are known, they are overriding. More often, considerations of quality of life become important in situations where the patient is incompetent to make decisions and no preference has been voiced previously. Economic considerations are becoming more and more important as health care resources become more scarce and decisions are made about the rationing and allocation of health care dollars. These considerations are very important in expensive, high-technology measures such as organ transplant and intensive care.

The physician's preferences are relatively unimportant in ethical decisions. Objective medical judgment is a critical input as described above, but subjective preference of the physician yields consistently to the patient's preference. However, physicians need not be compelled to act in ways contrary to their own ethical beliefs. For example, an obstetrician cannot be forced to perform abortions or an oncologist forced to provide ongoing chemotherapy for a patient with a terminal, end-stage illness. The physician does, however, have an obligation to assist a patient in finding a new provider who is able to work with the patient.

481. The answer is E. *(Pozgar, 4/e, pp 165–167.)* The Uniform Anatomical Gift Act permits persons 18 years of age or older to donate their body or parts of their body to medical education, science, or transplantation. The person must be of sound mind and the donation should be made by will or other written instrument. However, if the deceased has made no statements objecting to donation, a donation may still be made if relatives or guardians consent. This consent should be recorded. A donation may be revoked by written or oral means, with specific criteria for witnesses. Persons acting in good faith are not liable for criminal or civil negligence when participating in organ donation unless there has been notice of revocation of donation. This is designed to remove obstacles for participation in organ transplantation procedures and is similar to Good Samaritan laws. To eliminate conflict of interest and the overzealous harvesting of organs, time of death of the donor cannot be certified by any physician involved in the transplant procedure.

482. The answer is E. *(Jonsen, 2/e, pp 72–79.)* Requirements for competency to refuse or consent to medical treatment include attainment of legal age, the ability to comprehend and communicate information, and the ability to reason and deliberate about one's choices. The legal pronouncement may well require a judicial hearing, which may not be available in clinical emergencies. All the patients portrayed are presumed competent given the available information. Adherence to religious or unusual beliefs does not make one incompetent. Thus, the wishes of the Jehovah's Witness not to be transfused must be respected since they were expressed at a time when she was competent. Change in medical condition does not alter the power of the original statement. Similarly, affective states such as anxiety or (nonpathologic) depression do not make a patient incompetent when he or she refuses recommended medical treatment. One is ethically obligated to work with the patient in this situation and to try to explain options in a comforting manner, but patient autonomy still prevails. The elderly diabetic with a foot ulcer and the executive with chest pain are also competent to refuse medical treatment, for each is capable of understanding information and making a deliberate decision.

483. The answer is E. (*Pozgar 4/e, pp 28–29, 139–143.*) Physician-patient communication is considered confidential, but is not privileged to the extent of the attorney-client relationship. Violation of this confidentiality is termed *invasion of privacy* and can be cause for damages. However, physicians have specific legally defined reporting obligations, which include suspected child abuse, diseases in newborns, certain communicable diseases, births and deaths, suspicious deaths, and gunshot wounds (including those claimed to be accidental). When reporting these conditions in good faith, one is not liable for damages. Substance abuse, to the extent that it does not harm another person, is a confidential communication; such information should not be released without the patient's consent.

484. The answer is B. (*Pellegrino, JAMA 269:1158–1162, 1993.*) While Aristotle, Socrates, and Plato used medicine as a pedagogical tool, none produced a specific work on medical ethics. In addition to the items listed in the question, the Hippocratic Oath contains prohibitions against euthanasia and sexual relations with patients and exhorts the physician to a life of virtue. The prima facie principles include justice, autonomy, beneficence, and nonmaleficence. The ethics of caring do suggest that women are more caring in their ethical decisions; for example, they are more interested in reconciliation rather than in winning arguments. Clinical bioethics are not fully developed, but do provide for the empirical research and evaluation that any ethical system needs.

485. The answer is E. *(Dorland's Illustrated Medical Dictionary, 27/e, pp 767–768.)* Hippocrates (a late fifth century B.C. Greek) is often regarded as the "Father of Medicine." His oath emphasizes respect for teachers and the obligation to pass knowledge on to the next generation. It is the basis of the pledge to do only good and to do no harm. It specifically forbids active euthanasia, abortion, and the seduction of women or men "be they free or slaves." Substance abuse is not directly mentioned, although he swears "to preserve the purity of my life" and to "prescribe regimen for the good of my patient." Other medical oaths that contribute to the heritage of the physician's ethics include the Daily Prayer of Maimonides (a twelfth century Jewish physician and philosopher) and the Oath of Lasagna (a contemporary American physician).

486. The answer is C. *(Hulley, p 152.)* The DHHS does not require that subjects be compensated for their time or pain. However, some compensation may be helpful in recruiting adequate numbers of subjects for a study. Most importantly, the subjects must understand and must have given informed consent for any risk, inconvenience, or discomfort they will experience as a result of the study. Additional safeguards are required for vulnerable patients, such as prisoners, patients who are mentally incompetent, and children

487. The answer is C. *(Kircher, N Engl J Med 313:1263–1269, 1985.)* Because the information recorded on the death certificate is used in determining mortality from various diseases, it is essential that physicians understand how to fill one out. The immediate cause of death (in this case, pulmonary embolism) was not considered to be the condition that was responsible for the death by the attending physician, who determined that the patient died as a result of pancreatic cancer (which caused Trousseau's syndrome, which caused deep venous thrombosis, which resulted in a fatal pulmonary embolism). The last diagnosis listed is recorded in vital statistics; it should be the one that was responsible for setting in motion the eventually fatal chain of events.

488. The answer is D. *(Kircher, N Engl J Med 313:1163–1169, 1985.)* The death certificate has several purposes. It verifies that the patient died and gives the time and place of death and certain demographic information about the deceased. It also indicates the underlying disease that was responsible for the patient's death, so that accurate statistics on disease patterns can be kept. If there are reasons to be concerned about suspicious causes of death (such as poisoning), the physician should contact the coroner. In those cases, the coroner can

Can a woman … ord. autop ejn

pt's
final's
ms;hes

perform an autopsy at his judgment, even if the family refuses. In this case, as the patient's physician, you attended the death and have no reason to suspect foul play. Breast cancer was the disease that was responsible for her death and *must* be mentioned on the death certificate. Inclusion of the final conditions (cardiac tamponade, pericarditis) is optional. While there may be medical reasons to want an autopsy, it is inappropriate to refuse to sign a death certificate simply to force the family to acquiesce.

489–491. The answers are 489-D, 490-E, 491-B. *(Pozgar, 4/e, pp 38–39, 44, 81–82, 189–193.) Darling v. Charleston Community Memorial Hospital* (1965) established hospital liability for the actions of its employees. An 18-year-old football player fractured a leg, was treated in his local hospital over a 2-week period by a general practitioner without specialist consultation, subsequently developed complications, was transferred, and ultimately had a below-the-knee amputation. The physician settled out of court, but the case against the hospital continued with charges of negligence on a number of grounds, including failure to provide a sufficient number of trained nurses and failure of the nurses to bring the patient's condition to the attention of hospital officials so adequate consultation could be obtained. The hospital was found negligent and liable, thereby establishing the hospital's responsibility for the quality of the patient care administered in the institution. This also established the hospital's responsibility to monitor the credentials and competency of physicians.

The Quinlan case (1976) established that a patient's right to self-determination—and thus to decline medical treatment under certain situations—is protected by the right to privacy. The case involved a 21-year-old woman in a comatose vegetative state whose parents petitioned for the right to refuse treatment and turn off a respirator. The court reached its decision by balancing the state's interest in promoting the sanctity of life against the patient's privacy interest. The father was appointed legal guardian and in accordance with the findings of the hospital ethics committee, the respirator was turned off. Decisions regarding the withdrawal of life support remain very charged and controversial. Clear legal guidelines are still lacking for these decisions and individual decisions need to be made in each case with input from clinicians, ethicists, and often the courts.

Tarasoff v. Regents of the University of California (1976) confirmed the duty to warn. In the course of a psychotherapy session, a therapist was informed of a patient's intention to kill another person. The therapist failed to inform the victim of the patient's intentions, and the victim was subsequently murdered. The court held that the patient's right to privacy did not obviate the therapist's duty to warn possible victims in cases in which a therapist can *reasonably* determine that another person is at *foreseeable* risk. Performance of this duty may include notification of the police.

492–494. The answers are 492-C, 493-A, 494-D. *(Pozgar, 4/e, pp 23–25, 59–60.)* Abandonment is the unilateral termination of a doctor-patient relationship by the physician. It occurs when a physician terminates medical care prematurely (such as failing to follow up after an acute illness), fails to provide adequate cross-coverage, or refuses to see an established patient without notifying the patient and making arrangements to transfer care. The doctor-patient relationship may be ended by mutual consent of both parties, dismissal of the physician by the patient, absence of a requirement for continued medical care, or withdrawal of the physician with notification of the patient. This notification should be written and provide a reasonable transition period.

An assault is a threat to do harm. Battery involves touching another person in a socially unacceptable way without the person's consent. When informed consent is not obtained for medical procedures—diagnostic or therapeutic—battery is committed. The fact that the act may have improved the patient's health is legally irrelevant.

False imprisonment is the illegal confinement or restraint of a person or the illegal restraint of a person's liberty. A competent person who is not allowed to sign out against medical advice or who endures excessive use of physical restraints could sue for false imprisonment. Separate laws govern the involuntary hospitalization of the mentally ill.

495–497. The answers are 495-E, 496-A, 497-D. *(Jonsen, 2/e, pp 11–12, 47–51, 129–130, 141–142.)* Utilitarianism is the principle of doing the most good for the most people. It is useful in considering larger policy issues such as allocation of resources, but also applies to individual clinical decisions because in situations where resources are limited, providing care for one person may well mean denying care for another. As a general rule, preventive care will produce greater utility per unit of medical care than will intensive care.

Autonomy is the competent person's moral right to select his or her own course of action; it is a caveat of medical ethics. The corresponding legal principle is self-determination. A competent person may refuse life-sustaining care and those wishes must be respected. Paternalistic behavior—that is, performing actions in a person's best interests against his or her wishes—is ethically and legally permissible only in very limited situations. The case of the AIDS patient's refusal of intubation illustrates a decision not to progress to further intervention in a fatal disease. It is not an example of "passive" euthanasia, the withdrawal of life-sustaining therapy; nor is it an example of "active" euthanasia, the administration of a lethal agent to end suffering.

A supererogatory act is one beyond the call of duty—one that is morally praiseworthy but cannot be required of a person. No one can claim a corresponding right to the performance of this act. Organ donation, stopping at roadside emergencies, or providing patients with a home phone number could all be acts of supererogation, albeit in decreasing order of importance.

Beneficence is the principle "to do good." Along with nonmaleficence, "to do no harm," it is one of the cornerstones of medical ethics.

498–500.   The answers are 498-A, 499-C, 500-C. (*Pozgar, 4/e, pp 203–213.*) Professional liability insurance policies (malpractice coverage) include provisions for an insurance agreement, defense and settlement, the policy period, the amount payable, and the conditions of the policy. The policy period varies according to the type of insurance policy. An *occurrence* policy covers all incidents that take place during the year the policy is in effect, regardless of when they are reported or when legal action is initiated (given that the statute of limitations has not expired). Advantages of this form of insurance include continued coverage beyond the time period during which premiums are paid. For example, under this type of policy a retired physician would still be covered for events that occurred during active practice. In contrast, the *claims-made* policy covers only those claims made or reported during the policy year. Insurance companies worry about assuming liability for events that occurred prior to the initiation of the policy, and physicians must worry about ongoing coverage after the policy expires.

Malpractice policies cover professional liability only and contain limitations on the amount of damages covered. Policies usually contain a maximum for any individual claim as well as a limit to aggregate claims. Amounts awarded in excess of the insurance limit must be provided for by the individual professional. The insurance company agrees to provide a defense for the insured against lawsuits in which the attorney's obligations are to the insured professional directly, not to the insurance company. However, insurance companies often retain the power to effect a settlement, in which cases the attorney has responsibilities to the insurance company as well.

All insurance policies contain important provisions with which the physician must comply to keep the policy in effect, regardless of the policy period. These include requirements for prompt notification of occurrence and claim and a duty to assist the insurance company to reach a settlement. Other provisions govern relationships with other insurance companies, shared liability, and the terms of change or cancellation of the policy.

Bibliography

Behrman RE, Vaughan VC III: *Nelson Textbook of Pediatrics*, 14/e, Philadelphia, WB Saunders, 1992.

Benenson AS (ed): *Control of Communicable Disease in Man*, 15/e. Washington, DC, American Public Health Association Publications, 1990.

Browner WS, Newman TB: Are all significant p values created equal? The analogy between diagnostic tests and clinical research. *JAMA* 257:2459–2463, 1987.

Colton T: *Statistics in Medicine*. Boston, Little, Brown, 1975.

Dorland's Illustrated Medical Dictionary, 27/e. Philadelphia, WB Saunders, 1988.

Ehrlich O, Brem AS: A prospective comparison of urinary tract infections in patients treated with either clean intermittent catheterization or urinary diversion. *Pediatrics* 70:665, 1982.

Gray BH, McNerney MHA: For-profit enterprise in health care: The Institute of Medicine study. *N Engl J Med* 314:1523–1528, 1986.

Greaves WL, OrensteinWA, Hinman AR, et al: Clinical efficacy of rubella vaccine. *Pediatr Infect Dis* 2:284–286, 1983.

Green LW, Anderson CL: *Community Health*, 6/e. St. Louis, CV Mosby, 1990.

Hoekelman RA, Blatman S, Friedman SB, et al: *Primary Pediatric Care*. St. Louis, CV Mosby, 1987.

Hulley SB, Cummings S (eds): *Designing Clinical Research: An Epidemiologic Approach*. Baltimore, Williams & Wilkins, 1988.

Ingelfinger JA, Mosteller F, Thibodeau LA, Ware JH: *Biostatistics in Clinical Medicine*, 2/e. New York, Macmillan, 1987.

Jonsen AR, Siegler M, Winslade WJ: *Clinical Ethics*, 2/e. New York, Macmillan, 1986.

Kaplan H, Sadock J: *Comprehensive Textbook of Psychiatry*, 5/e. Baltimore, Williams & Wilkins, 1989.

Kircher T, Nelson J, Burdo H: The autopsy as a measure of accuracy of the death certificate. *N Engl J Med* 313:1263–1269, 1985.

Last JM (ed): *A Dictionary of Epidemiology*, 2/e. New York, Oxford University Press, 1988.

Last JM: *Maxcy-Rosenau Preventive Medicine and Public Health*, 13/e. East Norwalk, CT, Appleton & Lange, 1992.

Last JM: *Public Health and Human Ecology*. East Norwalk, CT, Appleton & Lange, 1987.

Levit KR, Lazenby HC, Cowan CA, Letsch SW: National health expenditures, 1990. *Health Care Financing Rev* 13:29–54, 1992.

Mausner JS, Kramer S: *Mausner and Bahn Epidemiology: An Introductory Text*, 2/e. Philadelphia, WB Saunders, 1985.

Michael M, Boyce WT, Wilcox AJ: *Biomedical Bestiary: An Epidemiologic Guide to Flaws and Fallacies in the Medical Literature*. Boston, Little, Brown, 1985.

Neinstein LS: *Adolescent Health Care: A Practical Guide*, 2/e. Baltimore, Urban & Schwarzenberg, 1991.

Nelson JD: *Pocketbook of Pediatric Antimicrobial Therapy*, 10/e. Baltimore, Williams & Wilkins, 1994.

Office of National Cost Estimates: National health expenditures. 1988. *Health Care Financing Rev* 11:1–41, 1990.

Pellegrino ED: The metamorphosis of medical ethics. *JAMA* 269:1158–1162, 1993.

Pozgar GD: *Legal Aspects of Health Care Administration*, 4/e. Rockville, MD, Aspen, 1990.

Relman AS: The new medical-industrial complex. *N Engl J Med* 303:963–970, 1980.

Rosenstock L, Cullen MR: *Clinical Occupational Medicine*. Philadelphia, WB Saunders, 1986.

Rothman KJ: *Modern Epidemiology*. Boston, Little, Brown, 1986.

Rudolph AM, et al (eds): *Pediatrics*, 18/e. East Norwalk, CT, Appleton & Lange, 1987.

Sackett DL, Haynes RB, Tugwell P: *Clinical Epidemiology: A Basic Science for Clinical Medicine*. Boston, Little, Brown, 1985.

Sanford JP: *Guide to Antimicrobial Therapy*. Dallas, Antimicrobial Therapy, Inc. 1993.

Schlesselman JJ, Stolley PD: *Case Control Studies: Design, Conduct, Analysis.* New York, Oxford University Press, 1982.

Siegel AF: *Statistics and Data Analysis: An Introduction.* New York, John Wiley & Sons, 1988.

United States Department of Health and Human Services (USDHHS): *Healthy People 2000: National Health Promotion and Disease Prevention Objectives.* Washington, DC, 1988.

United States Preventive Services (USPS) Task Force: *Guide to Clinical Preventive Services: An Assessment of the Effectiveness of 169 Interventions.* Baltimore, Williams & Wilkins, 1989.

Williams SJ, Torrens PR (eds): *Introduction to Health Services,* 4/e. New York, John Wiley & Sons, 1988.

Wilson JD, Braunwald E, Isselbacher KJ, et al (eds): *Harrison's Principles of Internal Medicine,* 12/e. New York, McGraw-Hill, 1991.

Wyngaarden JB, Smith LH Jr: *Cecil Textbook of Medicine,* 19/e. Philadelphia, WB Saunders, 1988.